Greg de Moore is an Associate Professor of Psychiatry based at Sydney's Westmead Hospital. He is the author of the bestselling *Tom Wills* and a co-author of *A National Game*. Greg has also written on the need to preserve psychiatric records as a precious storehouse of clinical and social history.

Ann Westmore is a Fellow in the Health Humanities and Social Science Unit, School of Population and Global Health at the University of Melbourne. Her PhD focused on psychiatry in mid-twentieth century Victoria.

GW00650243

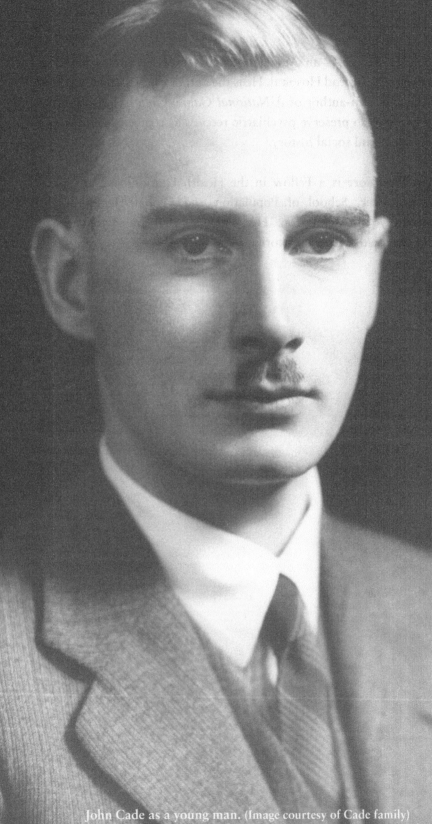

John Cade as a young man. (Image courtesy of Cade family)

Finding Sanity

John Cade, lithium *and the* taming *of* bipolar disorder

GREG DE MOORE *and* ANN WESTMORE

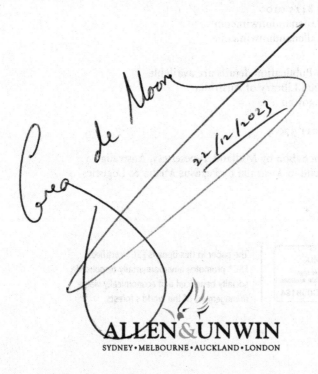

ALLEN&UNWIN
SYDNEY·MELBOURNE·AUCKLAND·LONDON

Allen & Unwin
83 Alexander Street
Crows Nest NSW 2065
Australia
Phone: (61 2) 8425 0100
Email: info@allenandunwin.com
Web: www.allenandunwin.com

Cataloguing-in-Publication details are available
from the National Library of Australia
www.trove.nla.gov.au

ISBN 978 1 76011 370 4

Set in 10.5/15 pt Sabon by Midland Typesetters, Australia
Printed and bound in Australia by Pegasus Media & Logistics

10 9 8 7 6 5 4

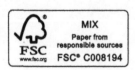

The paper in this book is FSC® certified.
FSC® promotes environmentally responsible,
socially beneficial and economically viable
management of the world's forests.

Contents

CONTENTS

*To my wife, Heather, and my children, Eve and Willem, for their
continued love and support during the research and writing of this
book. To my mother, Eileen, for planting in me a love of study.
To Ann and her family for helping complete this biography.
To the many wonderful mental health nurses with whom
I have worked over the years, in particular to the nurses of
the Bega Mental Health Unit.*
Greg de Moore

*To David and my extended family for their support and
encouragement, and to Greg and his family for aiding and abetting
the development and completion of this project.*
Ann Westmore

e question of scrap iron for Japan, right any he

was going to be done with it.

that this Indonesian bid for independence is only

head dissatisfaction by the peoples of the East over

ver lordship. The same problem is demanding solu

Burma and Indo China

of political speculation. Regarding leave, dea

ut at 28 days immediately following disembar

k or so in a convalescent camp (probably at Bal

over-haul, followed by another 30 days leave

are not sure of yet is whether we will get i

cumulated recreation leave which would amo

70-80 days. I suppose the department will

me as soon as possible - well, they will have

and I, darling, are entitled to a pretty good

that, I feel so rusty medically, that I simp

if possible three months post-graduate stud

like to do a month at St Vincents, a month at

a fortnight at the Eye and Ear, leaving ano

swinging - all provided we can keep the depa

then to work - as you guessed in one of your l

old brain box is simmering with ideas. I be

eriod of waiting has allowed many of my no

try to crystallise, and I'm just bursting to p

test. If they work out, they would represent a

the knowledge I've

Prologue

On a summer's day in early 1948, Edward sat alone, perched on the edge of the Sydney Harbour Bridge. For two hours he stared at the water below and contemplated what to do next.

Earlier the same day Edward had walked along Bondi Beach and conceived the idea of counting every grain of sand on the beach. It was part of his majestic plan—to sell off Bondi Beach, grain by grain. He figured that this would make him close to the richest man in the world. Of course, it was all part of Edward's delusional fantasy that summer's day. But to Edward it was all real; he just couldn't get this across to anyone.

Edward was suffering from mania, as part of his mental illness. He'd had this illness—manic depression, also known as bipolar illness or disorder—for nearly twenty years. He knew the inside of hospitals in and around Sydney and Melbourne well. And they knew him.

For weeks in early 1948 he'd been high, sky-rocket high, in the thick of a month-long manic episode; it was sweet and exhilarating. Selling Bondi Beach was just the latest of his many magnificent obsessions. He was known for them. Once, for example, he wrote a string of impassioned letters to the King of England seeking permission to construct a new naval base in Sydney Harbour. No answer was received from the Royals. Edward set about construction anyway, until the police picked him up. Another time he'd boasted of having invented a new type of engine to sell to General Motors Holden but nothing came of that either. Sometimes he hit the grog to slow things down, when words flowed furiously from his lips and he couldn't plug them. And this time Edward knew he was on a winner: selling Bondi Beach, now surely there'd be something in that.

As he took one final stroll along Bondi, he sensed the manic high and exaltation of the previous weeks start to fade; and in its place Edward felt the black chill of depression seep into his body. It was the first glimpse of a dark expanse he knew so well. The swing from high to low mood is the calling card of bipolar disorder. That's when Edward left the beach and made his way across town to the city's signature structure, the Sydney Harbour Bridge.

Edward believed that—if he survived the day—he would continue to live his life in and out of asylums, accumulating life's wreckage around him. In 1948, there was no effective medication for bipolar disorder. But while Edward sat and contemplated taking his life, something was taking place nearly 1000 kilometres away that would offer him a glimmer of hope. In that year, an Australian doctor, John Cade, discovered a treatment that has become the gold standard for bipolar disorder—lithium.

John Cade changed the course of medicine with his discovery of lithium; yet most doctors have never heard of him. His discovery has stopped more people from committing suicide than a thousand helplines, yet few counsellors know his name. And it has saved hundreds of billions of dollars in health care costs—enough to rival a nation's economy—but you can bet that no politician has the slightest idea of who John Cade was.

Lithium is the penicillin story of mental health. It was the first effective medication discovered for the treatment of a mental illness, and it is, without doubt, Australia's greatest mental health story.

Back in the summer of 1948, as Edward sat on the Sydney Harbour Bridge, wondering whether to jump, he could not have known that the world was on the cusp of a discovery that might change his life, and change the lives of the millions of 'Edwards' around the world, all sitting on their own bridges, and offer them a fighting chance in life. As it turned out, Edward stepped down from the bridge and returned to safety; many others over the years did not.

This is a book about a singular man, John Cade, and how he came upon a treatment that changed the face of medicine.

To start to understand that man, we have to go back to early in the twentieth century, to a small town in country Victoria. That's where the John Cade story takes flight.

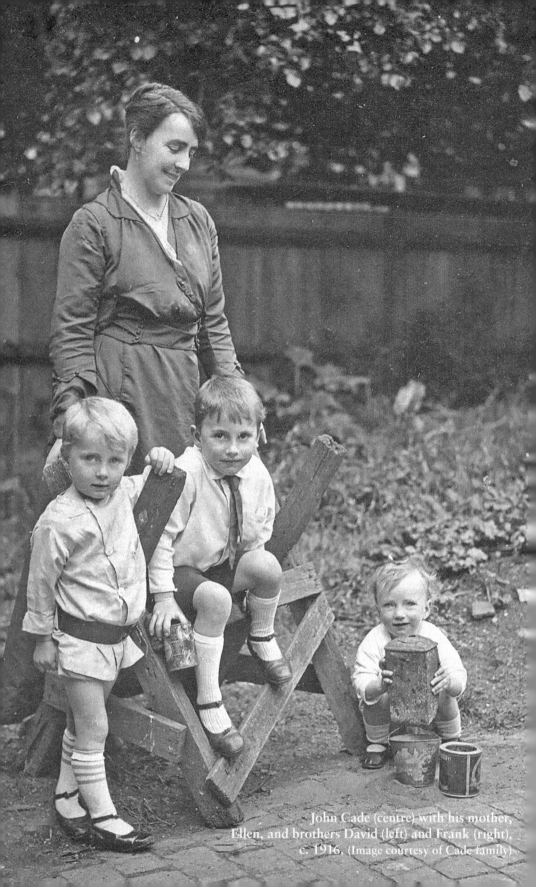

John Cade (centre) with his mother, Ellen, and brothers David (left) and Frank (right), c. 1916. (Image courtesy of Cade family)

PART 1

Playing ball
with Jesus

THE DISEASE:
Manic Depressive Insanity

As a rule the disease runs its course in isolated attacks ... we distinguish first of all *manic states* ... and *melancholia or depressive states* ... These two opposed phases of the clinical state have given the disease its name.

> '*Manic-Depressive Insanity*'
> *Emil Kraepelin, 1921*

...e question of scrap iron for Japan, right any h...
...was going to be done with it.

...that this Indonesian bid for independence is only...
...read dissatisfaction by the peoples of the East wi...
...ver lordship. The same problem is demanding solu...
...Burma and Indo china

...s of political speculation. Regarding leave, dea...
...ut at 28 days immediately following disembar...
...k or so in a convalescent camp (probably at Bal...
...l over-haul, followed by another 30 days leave
...are not sure of yet is whether we will get i...
...cumulated recreation leave which would amo...
...70-80 days. I suppose the department will
...me as soon as possible - well, they will have
...and I, darling, are entitled to a pretty good
...that, I feel so rusty medically, that I simp...
...if possible three months post-graduate stud...
...like to do a month at St Vincents, a month at
...a fortnight at the Eye and Ear, leaving a no
...swinging - all provided we can keep the depar...
...her to work - as you guessed in one of your l...
...old brain box is simmering with ideas. I be...
...eriod of waiting has allowed many of my no...
...try to crystallise, and I'm just bursting to p...
...test. If they work out, they would represent a ...
...the knowledge I...

I

John Frederick Joseph Cade was born on 18 January 1912 at Nurse Carroll's private hospital in Roberts Avenue in the Victorian country town of Horsham.

Sometimes Christian names mean very little; a mother's or a father's fancy, or a compromise when partners can't agree. But in John's case, never has a triplet of forenames so completely defined the roots of a man. And it is in the full flowering of John's name—John Frederick Joseph Cade—that the ancestral trail can be traced, at least on the paternal side.

In order, he 'was named after his great-great-grandfather, great-grandfather and grandfather', so John's father proudly wrote. The names of John, Frederick and Joseph were the first names of a string of male Cades dating back to late eighteenth-century England—nearly all were medical men or pharmacists, a near unbroken line of chemists and doctors breeding true for close to 150 years. And of these forebears, it was Frederick Cade, born in 1802, who migrated from England to the Antipodes, putting down roots in a very youthful Melbourne and establishing one of the earliest pharmacies in the fashionable east end of Collins Street. We can find Frederick Cade's name as a 'druggist' at 134 Collins Street, Melbourne, from 1842, just seven years after John Batman signed a treaty with Wurundjeri Aboriginal people and the site was settled.

John's birth, as far as we know, was without incident. Certainly his father, Dr David Cade, had taken pains to make sure that a trusted colleague, a Dr Read, resident in Horsham, was present as Ellen gave birth to their first child. David Cade, however, was not present—the norm for husbands at the time—presumably doing his rounds as a country doctor. As for Nurse Carroll, she assisted Dr Read in bringing John Cade into the world.

Nurse Carroll's private hospital was one of several private hospitals in Horsham in the early twentieth century. A beautiful timber building with luxuriant palms and large pine trees in the front garden, it has long since gone, replaced by a motel. The only thing of beauty and substance remaining from the original hospital are two tall pine trees standing in the bitumen carpark of the motel; trees, rather than distinguished and beautiful old buildings, seemingly more immune to a developer's wallet.

Several faded black and white photographs exist of this early twentieth-century private hospital. They show a small hospital, actually more like a large gracious home with two decorated timber gables overlooking the front garden than a hospital. In one photo, three nurses stand erect in the garden dressed head to toe in glowing white fabric, like a vision from heaven. Nurses to whom you'd entrust your baby's and wife's health.

Just before the birth of his first child, we find Dr David Cade highlighted in the local *Horsham Times* newspaper. It reported on 16 January 1912 that David Cade was urgently summoned to attend the one-eyed Reverend Hillier who, in the midst of a church service, dramatically lost all sight in his good eye. Apparently, this blackout took place as the service was ending, just after the benediction and before amen. Whilst David Cade was tending him, the reverend's sight miraculously returned. Whether this was a case of divine intervention or the healing powers of a country general practitioner is not quite clear. Not being an assiduous churchgoer himself, David Cade may have preferred an explanation that credited his medical skills while his wife, Ellen, a fervent Catholic, may have given more weight to spiritual factors. If nothing else, it was the best of omens. For two days later Ellen gave birth to a healthy son.

———

Some of John Cade's personality traits clearly sprang from his medical father. But he owed at least one important characteristic to his mother. And, in the end, that single dimension may have been the most vital attribute of all: tenacity. Without it even the most talented man falls short. Family stories recall a tough, thick-skinned and determined woman. Well before her marriage, Ellen Edwards showed plenty of character:

> As a younger woman she was fierce. She was one of those strong pioneer-type women. A reasonably tall woman, she was phys-ically strong. I remember a story of a time when she went to collect eggs from the hen house. She'd been losing a few eggs and she thought the culprit might have been a fox; but when she went in there was a rat in the chook pen. She saw this rat and quick as a flash she grabbed it by the tail and slung it on the timber post.

Originally from Clunes, near Ballarat, Ellen Edwards was a trained nurse and gained appointments to a string of country hospitals in New South Wales and Victoria. In 1896 the *Goulburn Evening Penny Post* reported that a Miss Edwards of Bathurst had been appointed assistant nurse at Narrandera, in the Riverina region of southern New South Wales.

By 1903 she was contending with a typhoid outbreak in Condobo-lin, where she was matron. Later the same year, at a farewell at Condobolin Hospital, a large number of friends and well-wishers heard the mayor praise her to the rafters for her contribution to the central NSW community among whom she had lived for the previous six years. He commended her 'kind attention to all who had come under her care', adding that by her 'genial manner, she had endeared herself to all'. The local Justice of the Peace intoned that the hospital had never had a more conscientious matron. She was showered with presents from the hospital committee. But what impressed the local newspaper even more was the gift of a lady's handbag from a Miss Gertie Simpson, a former patient who simply wanted to express her gratitude to the departing matron.

Nurse Ellen Edwards was a substantial woman from all accounts: straight-backed and broad at the shoulders. For Ellen to succeed in nursing it helped to have a strong back and broad shoulders, particularly in country hospitals where access to attendants was limited. Although accustomed to running her own show, when Ellen gained appointment to Mildura Hospital in northern Victoria in 1904 she was third in charge. But typhoid once again struck and ten people died, including members of the senior nursing staff. So Ellen was soon appointed matron. By 1905 her repute was such that nearby Balranald Hospital enticed her to join, and while working there she met David Cade, who had recently bought into a general practice in the town.

Three years later the pair married in the Catholic Cathedral in Bendigo. There was no talk of David, who had been brought up in the Church of England, converting to Catholicism. But it is likely, in accordance with Catholic ecclesiastical tradition, he agreed that any children would be raised as Catholics. Ellen Edwards was a hard-bitten Catholic and her Irish Catholic heritage was a matter of great pride to her. But as one of her future daughters-in-laws was to slyly remark when asked about Ellen's religion: 'She was a devout Catholic when it suited her.'

When John, her first child, came into the world, a resolute Ellen Cade (née Edwards)—rat killer and Catholic—kept a sharp eye on her newborn son.

Not a great deal is known of John's first few years. His father simply stated, as if observing John purely from a scientific standpoint, that his firstborn 'developed satisfactorily and made steady progress mentally and physically during his first year of life'. Some years later David Cade, through that same detached lens, cut to the core of his son's temperament: 'In his infancy he was a strange mixture of gravity and brightness and quite early he manifested signs of that spirit of investigation and experimentation.'

On one memorable morning, while Ellen was attending Mass and David was having a sleep-in, John gave his father a terrible shock by inserting something into his father's ear canal, seemingly endeavouring to find out more about it. Jumping up, his startled father told him to desist, but John was soon at it again.

From the very beginnings of his life, he was a child whose logical manner, curiosity and persistence impressed observers. John Cade, whatever else his attributes, was born with a tidy, tenacious and inquisitive mind.

––––––

Although he was born in the rural town of Horsham, about 300 kilometres northwest of Melbourne, if you journey there you won't find much evidence of John's existence, or indeed of the Cade family history. For that you need to take a short pilgrimage of another 30 kilometres to the smaller town of Murtoa, where John's father—Dr David Cade—was the local general practitioner, and where the Cade family lived.

When you get to Murtoa, there is no way you can miss the Memorial Archway—right next to the splendid lake in the town's centre. Just about every country town in Australia boasts a similar memorial, listing all the local men and women who fought in the First and Second World Wars. Rarely do people take the time to look closely, but if you run your eyes down the column of names for the Great War, about halfway down you will come to the name of Dr David Duncan Cade chiselled into the granite. When the First World War broke out, Dr David Cade enlisted; before long he was heading to Europe.

––––––

In 1915, David Cade left his country practice in Murtoa to fight for 'King and Country'. The 40-year-old country doctor, already a veteran of the Boer War, was imbued with the deepest sense of patriotism, and when the First World War ignited he readily signed up. On his departure from Australia he left his wife, Ellen, and three young boys to do their best in the circumstances; John, the oldest, was just three years of age.

David Cade spent four dark and disturbing years in Gallipoli and France. On one occasion, anticipating a Turkish assault, he prepared for the inevitable casualties—setting out bandages, stretchers and all the accoutrements a doctor at war might need. When he looked up from the neat piles of white cloth that lay before him, he observed 'a young soldier carrying a petrol tin of water for a machine gun' rushing past, 'but he had hardly gone five or ten yards further when an enemy shell came up the valley and carried his head away'. David Cade records this in a matter-of-fact manner, implicitly understanding that embellishment could only detract from its telling.

At another time, near the village of Pozières, in France, he recalls 'a German who was wounded in No-Man's Land and brought in after four days' with a 'leg smashed above the knee' and 'stinking horribly'. Festering bacteria would normally bloat the leg with gas gangrene—an ominous portent for any soldier—but on this occasion David Cade noted with a deep curiosity the absence of the toxic, swelling gas. As he separated the folds of rotting flesh in the German's leg, both doctor and patient observed a writhing mass of maggots in the congealed blood, the stench of dead meat terrific. A dispassionate David Cade dismembered the soldier's leg using a 'butcher's amputation' and, although we never learn what this exactly entailed, it sounds sufficiently gruesome and descriptive to appreciate that no great sophistication was involved. The following day, the now one-legged German soldier awoke, apparently much improved and ravenous to boot. He turned and politely asked his captors for a sausage. We can only hope it was duly given.

Not long before war's end, while stationed in France, David Cade recorded how a boyish-looking soldier prepared to take off a backpack. Without warning, a shard of shrapnel from an exploding shell pierced the boy's chest; death was instant. Cade, who was standing nearby, was spared, unhurt. Years afterwards, David Cade recalled how he looked upon this young man lying in the mud, mesmerised by the youth's untouched face, now drained of life. That image of innocence—angelic, white and dead—never left David Cade.

When he returned to Australia in 1919, it was with an urgency to make up for lost time and reunite with his family. Waiting were his wife and three sons, John, David and Frank. John was the only one of the three boys who had any memories of their father. Now seven, the youngster had changed a great deal over the previous four years, but so had his father. War badly scarred David Cade's mind; he was not the same man who set forth from Australia, Gallipoli-bound, in 1915. David Cade is not remembered as a warm or affectionate man, but rather as austere and fusty, any softer attributes having been stripped away by war. If any one of his children were to have noticed the change, it would have been his eldest, John.

2

While David Cade was away at war, Ellen and the three boys moved from Murtoa to a succession of boarding houses in the cool-climate country on the outskirts of northeast Melbourne, counting out pennies to each new landlady. When David returned from war, he was keen to see his eldest son, but from the start theirs would be a formal relationship. Although there was deep affection between them, John only ever called his father 'sir'. This, no doubt, was expected of boys of his generation, but it was also a social grace that allowed any complicating emotions between father and son never to interfere.

After returning from the First World War, David Cade appraised his own life as a 'failure'. On more than one occasion he wrote of lost opportunities. Yet to read his letters and the memoir he penned in 1945 (about his observations on life and art), and to ponder his courageous exploits during war, we can be in no doubt that here was a highly intelligent and brave man, with perceptive and well-informed views; however, he despaired over his life and continually berated himself for his self-described failings. Ambition called him but he felt unable to respond. This preoccupation with perceived failure in all likelihood points to David Cade's psychological wounds from the war. His visions of dead and dying men didn't dissolve, no matter how hard friends and family might have wished those visions away or just, mistakenly, assumed their disappearance over time. David Cade diagnosed himself as having 'war-weariness'; others called it 'shellshock' but today we would call it post-traumatic stress disorder. Titles change; the symptoms don't. Whatever fashionable label we use, David Cade was as much a victim of war as the boys he saw cut down around him. When he returned to country Victoria he felt unable to cope with the trials of daily house calls and the relentless demands of general practice.

Instead, he sought refuge from the mental anguish of incessant general practice and applied for a position as a doctor in an asylum for the insane—hoping for a regular government salary and less stress. So, like the refugee from war he was, David Cade took a medical post with the Lunacy Department in the small, pretty town of Beechworth in northeastern Victoria's alpine country.

In 1920, David, accompanied by Ellen and the three boys, moved to the Beechworth Hospital for the Insane. The Cade family settled into a doctor's cottage in the grounds of the hospital, and for the next two years, the asylum—with its towering walls, farm and garden, set high above the township—was home. As late as the 1990s, an ex-nursing staff member of Beechworth could recall stories of the doctor and young John walking the asylum grounds together.

The period from eight to ten years of age is an impressionable one for a boy—a time when ideas and dreams take root in his mind; an uncomplicated time he will look upon for the remainder of his life. In 1920, a typical eight-year-old boy played cricket with his mates on the streets of suburban Melbourne; John played games in a lunatic asylum with disturbed men who thought they were Jesus. There can be little doubt that in these germinal years John's affection for the mentally ill stirred and took root.

In 1922 Dr David Cade and his family transferred from Beechworth to the northern outskirts of Melbourne, to the Sunbury Asylum for the Insane. The Cades remained there only a short time. A government archive—a school register—in one thin, erratic scribble, places John and his brothers at the local Sunbury State School for a handful of months. There is a paucity of personal reflections at this part of the story and few official records to enlighten us. But we do know from family lore that, as a boy, John was a collector—of stones, of insects and of words. And he was a classifier, carefully placing everything into columns and rows in the same way that a nineteenth-century naturalist might, and labelling everything neatly and precisely. John displayed an innate and joyous curiosity, and early on exhibited a love of the natural world. There was a compulsiveness to it all—picking up a stone to investigate its geology, fully prepared for some secretive creature lurking beneath in its shadow; it was a thoroughness he brought to everything he did.

In 1922, after their short stint at the Sunbury Asylum, the family moved again, this time to the more modern and spacious Mont Park Hospital for the Insane located at the intersection of suburban Heidelberg, Macleod and Bundoora.

Although the dates are unclear we know that John attended the local Heidelberg State School along with a new mate, Bennie Rank. John and Bennie became part of a small select group of pupils offered tuition by the headmaster, Mr Frank Clough, for scholarships aiming (we imagine) at more prestigious schools. As it turned out, neither John nor Bennie won scholarships, but this was the first time others marked John out for exceptional treatment and possible higher honours in life.

After school each day John practised tennis, hitting balls for hours against a high brick wall of one of the Mont Park Asylum wards; or he carted a set of clubs across Plenty Road for a game of golf with his mother, or brother David, both golf fanatics; John, whatever the sport, was blessed with adroit hand–eye coordination. While tennis in particular was a passion, boxing was a necessity for self-defence. Boxing for a boy in the mid-1920s was as much a manly rite of passage as was a clumsy first shave. John was a keen student of pugilism and anointed himself as the guardian of his two younger brothers. Bullying, far from a modern curse, lurked nearby and threatened the younger pair, so John became their protector. Like so much in his early life he learned the craft of boxing from an asylum patient, a 'dear old man' who pranced about Mont Park Hospital sparring—imitating the 1920s world heavyweight champ, Jack Dempsey—with invisible foes. We don't know any more about this insane instructor of John Cade, though we wish we did. Perhaps it was a psychotic patient, or an old soak—one of the many brain-damaged drunkards who'd dissolved their brains with booze—or a boxer with a scarred brain from the relentless accumulation of hits in a boxing tent. Who knows? But in the 1920s there was no shortage of such candidates to offer the young pugilist tuition. And John, apparently, was not shy in taking it up.

———

In 1925, John entered the exclusive Scotch College in leafy Hawthorn, Melbourne, a school favoured by some of the wealthiest families in Australia to educate their sons. An article published by the *Age* newspaper in 2010 noted that Scotch College, the second-oldest extant school in Victoria, boasted more honoured Australians among its alumni than any other school in the nation. In 1925 it had just enrolled one more future star.

The choice of Scotch College tells us something else about John: that he was a boy who thought for himself. When John's father—an Anglican—brokered an agreement with his Irish Catholic wife, allowing the children to be raised as Catholics, he insisted as a compromise that the boys be given the choice of their secondary school. John's father had gone to a prestigious Anglican School, Melbourne Grammar. And we would expect most sons would simply follow in their father's footsteps. But despite having an Anglican father and Catholic mother, John, in the finest ecumenical spirit, plumped for the Presbyterian school his grandfather Joseph had attended. To cap it off, John's enrolment form described his religion as Roman Catholic. Years later, John told his family that he felt somewhat 'on the outer' at Scotch, that in this Presbyterian School he had to prove to himself that his Catholic faith was soundly based.

Knowledge about John's time at Scotch College is sparse, gleaned largely from the memories of a few fellow students and the occasional line left to us in the school's yearbooks. He played Australian Rules football for his House, but not that well, and he was studious and meticulous about everything he did in the world of academia. Although clearly bright, there is no suggestion that he was a precocious student or marked out for future achievements any more than his fellow classmates. In his final year he excelled in biology, taking first-class honours and he also did well in chemistry, physics and English, snaring third-class honours in all three.

It remains a long-held family belief that John's interest in and aptitude for chemistry goes back to Frederick Cade, who migrated to Australia in the 1840s and set up his pharmacy nearly a decade before the Victorian gold rush. The Cade family archives include a mottled photograph of Frederick—a stern, bearded figure with grizzled hair, a creased face and arms folded like a disapproving maths teacher. The first Cade to set foot in Melbourne looks like a man you'd rather not meet. But he is treasured among the family's amateur historians and his photograph is pulled reverentially from the family folder. John himself was proud of this connection with Frederick Cade the 'druggist' and of his own deep bloodlines that led directly to the birth of Melbourne and the start of colonial chemistry.

John remained at Scotch College, matriculating at the end of 1928. Turning over the pages of the various yearbooks there is a veritable acreage of names to plough through looking for the one name you really want to find—to uncover what John did or didn't do during those youthful years. And always looking for clues as to what might make this individual exceptional. Perhaps, in truth, we also scour these lines for ordinariness; to confirm our nascent belief that we all can achieve greatness regardless of the mediocrity of performance at school.

His name appears in these yearbooks among some other notables, and in the sea of students who drifted into and out of school, unrecognised and unrecognisable. Scotch nurtured a talented bunch in his year: Sir Archibald Glenn, industrialist and Managing Director of ICI (now Orica); Justice C.I. Menhennit of abortion law fame; C.D. Kemp, co-founder of the Institute of Public Affairs; E.R. Love, Professor of Pure Mathematics at the University of Melbourne; as well as E.A.H. Laurie, writer and communist advocate. And then there was Bennie Rank, John's tennis partner and co-catcher of trains to Flinders Street and on to Scotch College, who rose to head Plastic Surgery at Royal Melbourne Hospital, tucking a knighthood into his kit along the way.

In the archive folder the school keeps on John Cade, we found an unexpected black and white photograph. It shows John, in his Scotch regalia, with his father and younger brothers. This photo catches him between childhood and adulthood: the date is 1928, so John is sixteen. He lounges, languidly, with a semi-tropical palm behind him, as if stretched out on a deck chair beside a pool in a dreamy, decadent scene from *The Great Gatsby*; it is the sweet period before the world fell apart after the Great Stock Market Crash. On closer scrutiny John looks like he might be wearing his cricket creams beneath his school blazer; and, although not, should be sipping iced tea and consuming cucumber sandwiches. The school has labelled this 1928 photo with the less-than-illuminating title: 'Activity—Famous'.

John's father, on the other hand, looks uptight and fully buttoned-up in a three-piece suit. With a face as severe as Frederick Cade's, it is, perhaps, no wonder John only ever addressed his father as 'sir'.

At the end of school and with over 150 years of dynastic tradition and expectation, it hardly raised an eyebrow when—driven to succeed and talented to boot—John chose to study medicine at the University of Melbourne.

In 1929, John commenced the first of six years of his medical course. When his father returned to Beechworth that year as the asylum's medical superintendent, John remained in Melbourne and boarded with his aunt Rene in Orrong Road, Toorak, at five guineas rent per week. When it came to money, John had a scrupulous moral code. When his uncle, a general practitioner in the town of Narrabri, NSW, died in 1931 he left some money to John, who immediately used it to repay his own father for his medical education.

His fellow students remember John as an organised and careful student and were not surprised when he was awarded the forensic medicine prize in his final year. Benjamin Rank remembered that John was 'up in the top marks' and 'was research minded, keeping details and classifications' during their resident and postgraduate years. John's bosom pal at university and fellow Catholic, Frank Prendergast, concurred and also recalled John's fascination with all things 'biochemical', adding that John 'was always meticulous in everything he did'. Prendergast, who was to later study and practise psychiatry, saw John as a highly distinctive individual, a man who was 'rarely ruffled', and commented that beneath John's calm exterior he was never frightened of physical confrontation. Prendergast cited an incident when John was betrayed by an acquaintance; in a righteous rage, John exploded and summarily kicked the offending person 'in the backside'. It made an impression on Prendergast precisely because it was one of the few times he saw John's anger erupt.

It is part of Cade family lore how, at university, John boxed against Edward 'Weary' Dunlop, no slouch with the gloves himself and later one of Australia's most recognised Second World War heroes. And how John sparred with Bennie Rank, whose nose he flattened (very apt, considering Sir Benjamin rose to be one of Australia's most prominent plastic surgeons).

In the final year of his medical course, John attended twelve lectures on mental diseases. We have John's psychiatry textbook from that time, a slender maroon volume titled *Aids to Psychiatry* by William Siegfried Dawson, one of the first psychiatric professors appointed in Australia. It is the first time we come across John's signature style of scrupulously underlining sentences with the steadiest of hands, a clue to his character. If assiduous attention to detail is any indication of his approach to psychiatry then he, unlike so many of his fellow students, saw psychiatry as a subject worthy of serious study.

————————

John's first year as a doctor was spent at St Vincent's Hospital, the flagship Catholic hospital in Melbourne. The following year, having decided to study paediatrics, he worked at the Children's Hospital. By now his father had returned from Beechworth and was back at Sunbury Asylum. John returned to live with his parents and scooted back and forth between Sunbury and the Children's Hospital on his very stylish, newly purchased, English-made Francis-Barnett motorcycle. It was on one of these trips to the Children's Hospital that he became ill.

In 1936, antibiotics were unheard of and 'catching a chill' was the ominous phrase that parents uttered when one of their children fell ill. Without antibiotics this could be a death sentence. So it was with some anxiety that David Cade recalled John catching 'a chill in foul weather'. Within days John fell desperately ill with pneumococcal pneumonia and was confined to bed at the Children's Hospital. He was nursed around the clock; his parents—fearing the worst—expected him to die. John's father recalled the outlook when the infection spread from one to both lungs: 'His condition . . . appeared very grave and one Sunday morning . . . we had become certain that he would not survive the day.'

But survive the day he did; and at night a young, beautiful brunette nurse sat by his bedside and cared for him. Her name was Estana Evelyn Jean Charles, but everyone just called her Jean. A highly intelligent and warm woman who had gained certificates in three areas of nursing, she sponged John's body, switched on the oxygen cylinders that brought him life-giving gas, and, by the bedside, prayed for her patient.

Jean remembered: 'He came down with a very bad pneumo-
nia . . . I wasn't to turn him or move him unless I had permission . . .
he was very, very ill . . . the priest was called.'

When, against expectations, John's fever broke and his laboured
breathing eased, his father praised a 'merciful' god for his son's salvation. John lifted his weakened frame from the hospital bed and spent
time talking to his nurse, Jean; apparently, even in such sickness, he
liked what he saw. On the day he was discharged he came back and
asked her out to dinner.

Somewhere along the way, in a moment of epiphany, John abandoned the idea of becoming a paediatrician and decided to take up
his father's profession, psychiatry. In November 1936, John Cade,
now 24 years old, was duly appointed as a Medical Officer in the
Victorian Department of Mental Hygiene and headed off to Beechworth Mental Hospital, with his dog Bonzo the Fourth tagging
along for company.

3

Beechworth Hospital for the Insane opened in 1867. Even today the three-storey main building is gloomily impressive, and its parallel lines of deep-set windows, like empty eye sockets, brood over the acres of picturesque grounds below. Modelled on the grand English asylum plan devised by Dr John Conolly, its Italianate corridor-style buildings stand like a silent stone penitentiary. For nearly 130 years this site was a sink of insanity; one of a handful of places where much of the madness in the state of Victoria was corralled and condensed. Originally built for 400 patients, it often crammed closer to a thousand men and women behind its bluestone walls. It was constructed on the beautiful hills that overlook the township of Beechworth; everyone knew if you were heading 'up the hill' you were off to the asylum.

The hospital site, after 128 years, was decommissioned in 1995 as a psychiatric hospital. To stroll around the many acres now with its dozens of empty buildings is quite something. If you venture there in the first hour after sunrise, the air is sweet and clear; the dawn frost lies thick on the acres of grass that recede into the distance. It is one of the prettiest spots in the state of Victoria.

The freshness and clarity of the outside air is at odds with the dank and stifling gloom deep within the abandoned buildings. Inside, the echo of one's tread on the stone stairway is sharp; and the clank of each closing lock has a ring of ominous finality. Decrepit beauty abounds in these century-old buildings, even as the walls decay and paint flakes. This is a place calcified in time. Pigeons roost by the hundreds in the alcoves.

Outside, if you stand still for a moment, it is not hard to imagine the hospital in its heyday in the 1930s: the covered walkways, now empty, rattling and humming like a main street with workers pushing trolleys filled with laundry or meals from the kitchen; at the change of a twelve-hour shift, a pullulating mass of workers streaming down the hill, an equal number plying their way up the hill to the hospital. This crush of employees—earning a living and working in the hospital for the insane—breathed life into the economy of Beechworth.

Older nurses can still remember the terrific din of humanity in the asylum. The raucous and rowdy noise of around a thousand captive souls floated down the hill to the town, day and night.

Death was common in the asylum, especially in the colder months. Winter was an unforgiving time, and the shadows were deep and long; the chill air silently carried away dozens of patients each year. It was often a junior attendant or nurse who'd cart the dead from the ward to the mortuary. To do so in the dark of night was a rite of passage for new staff; the common initiation ritual was for older staff to spring out of the blackness to terrify the new nurse to see if he or she were made of stern-enough stuff.

The old hospital mortuary now stands in solitude. Painted white, it looks more like a public toilet block from a distance. By peering through a window, the slab where the dead rested is still visible. In a final insult to the faded grandeur of the old hospital, the depredation of vandals has taken its toll and graffiti daubs the once-beautiful stone walls, this defacement reflecting a different type of disturbed mind. Near the porter's gate, at the old entrance at the top of the hill, there is a flyer on the ground advertising ghost tours at night in the asylum: cheap thrills, no doubt, and a way to make a living for someone in the 21st century.

Myths and stories about the hospital still linger in the pubs and homes down the hill, and the Beechworth townsfolk still regale visitors with a repertoire of tales. Mrs Zwar was the young daughter of Dr Naylor, the psychiatrist superintendent of the asylum in the 1920s. She vividly remembered that one of the asylum doctors believed a full moon caused madness. The cautious doctor could be seen on bright nights on his nocturnal strolls between the hospital wards, umbrella aloft, shielding his cranium from the mind-damaging lunar beams.

This story, perhaps apocryphal, nonetheless hints at the medieval mindset of asylum life in late 1936, when 24-year-old John Cade having spent just a few months studying psychiatry, turned up for his first day within the stone walls of Beechworth.

———

John was warmly greeted by nurses who remembered his father and 'the young boy' from his time there in the early 1920s. Allocated a doctor's cottage, he settled in and spent his first night as a fully fledged asylum doctor.

'My first introduction to my new patients took place early on the morning after my arrival, as I was in the midst of a bath.'

From somewhere came the sharp-edged call: 'Do you keep a cat?' John answered in the negative.

'Then do you keep a dog?' As Bonzo the Fourth, John's canine companion, had accompanied him, he answered honestly.

'Can't stand cats or dogs. I'm leaving,' came the reprimand.

John, not certain where the questioner was located and curious about who they were, stepped out of the bath, dried himself, and assumed his 'professional dignity'. Rather than leaving, the interlocutor—'a thin misanthropic, elderly apparition with two front teeth missing'—was still present. 'She had evidently assumed, very conditionally, the position of housekeeper.' This was John's introduction to Mrs Arkins, his first Beechworth patient; she spent the better part of the day nosing about his cottage, making his bed and doing a little sweeping. Within no time his pyjamas were dashed off to the laundry, so he slept in his tennis shirt, and a general chaos engulfed his household.

Then there was the comical Ethel, who accosted John each
morning as he struck out from his cottage across the asylum grounds
to the locked wards:

> A gorgeous creature . . . like a coy bird of paradise . . . Ethel
> is seventy, short, uraemic, romantic, painted and panting. It
> starts something like this: 'Oh, dear doctor, you're so tall, so
> handsome, I knew your *darling* father (so kind to me, don't
> you know). My back is aching so, you will give me some more
> of that ginger mixture darling Dr Trembath ordered for me,
> won't you.'

A resplendent Ethel wore lips as scarlet as the reddest rose with
cheeks to match, and charcoal eyeliner; she was an apparition to
stop John in his tracks. Ethel, like a swaying temptress, danced
'coyly about me and would certainly embrace me but for the guard-
ianship of the matron and the nurse in charge of the ward. She is
terribly jealous and has retired to her room temporarily since I have
announced that I have decided to extract the two remaining front
teeth of her rival', a certain Mrs Cole.

John settled into this rural retreat of the deranged—a world
full of Ethels—and gulped in whatever goodness and knowledge he
could find. As for the institution, John was less than impressed. 'The
whole place is constructed on the idea that mentally afflicted people
are infinitely more dangerous than criminals, with no regard for
their comfort.' Some patients remained in the asylum, imprisoned,
for decades.

John immediately caused a stir when he announced to the matron
that he would like to do ward rounds and (heaven forbid) speak to
the patients. Hospital staff were not accustomed to such unortho-
dox and undoctorly habits; indeed, the matron retorted—with what
we imagine was an impatient air—John would only be required
to attend ward rounds when she alerted him to a problem. John

listened to this advice and then ignored it in a spirit of quiet insurrection: young Dr Cade set about seeing patients each day. And if this was a surprise to the sleepy attendants at Beechworth, well, they were in a veritable tizz when the young doctor physically examined his charges and dared open up their medical records to write his daily observations. At the time it was common for doctors' notes on patients to be brief or non-existent, other than for the initial interview or during episodes of acute ill-health. By providing a daily assessment, John and other staff members were better placed to observe and manage early signs of physical or mental deterioration or improvement. From the very start Dr Cade Jnr, unlike his father, was a revolutionary.

When John entered the locked wards of Beechworth, the first thing he noted was an acrid aroma—faeces smeared by patients into keyholes, and the unholy triad of stale urine, tobacco and floor polish. This swirling mix rose like fumes from the stinking bilge of a ship. Many patients looked downtrodden—socks scrunched around ankles and coats shabbily slipping from shoulders were a common sight; frumpy dresses were the rule. As one retired female nurse remarked when recalling this dull plumage: 'All the girls' clothing was made in the sewing room . . . the girls had blue and white striped dresses . . . it was awful. They had no underpants.' Toilet paper was a luxury; newspaper a convenient alternative. Seeking beauty, and just a bit of humanity, female patients crushed geranium petals as rouge for their cheeks, and sometimes styled their hair with cooking fat when soap was absent.

Outside the wards some patients perched on steps, others loped about, shuffling through the loose dirt like street sweepers. These abandoned individuals were the discarded detritus of Australian life. Visitors, and there were not many, gawked at their oddities. There were, of course, the usual assortment of asylum inmates—the melancholics rocking to a rhythm unheard; the paranoid patients plotting yet another revenge; the manics—frenetic and incoherent; the docile—vitality drained—ossified into an existence like the bluestone they sat on; and the occasional catatonic patient, stiff and seemingly uncomprehending, like an Easter Island statue.

Many nurses were remarkably caring; some were not. Taunting patients to provoke them was an awful game played by a few pernicious nurses to disrupt the boredom of a long day in the asylum. The staff anointed patients as either 'good' or 'difficult'. It was a functional, if crude, bifurcation. 'Good' patients, John recalled, 'were encouraged to assist in the wards by polishing and scrubbing floors, making beds, washing foul clothes and bed linen, and helping in the kitchen and dining room'. The 'good' patients helped crank the asylum to life every morning. 'Difficult' patients were another matter altogether. Aggressive types might be isolated in wooden cubicles several metres long and several metres wide; with a single split door like a horse stall. A sliding shutter opened in the top half to enable the attendant to view the patient.

Physical restraint was common, some patients trussed up like poultry and released only at feeding times. There was a repertoire of canvas restraints, which read like a department store catalogue—camisoles, vests, dresses and jackets, designed for men and women. All coarse and stiff like steel, appearing to be unfit for humans but used nonetheless.

Some patients openly masturbated; offending hands were placed into canvas muffs, which in turn were sewn tightly onto a canvas vest, wrapping the arms around the waist and rendering them immoveable. Not quite clapped in leg-irons, but not that different. Only an act of God, or a nursing attendant, could offer liberation.

All manner of patients were thrown into mental hospitals like Beechworth. Most were obviously sick, others were troublesome, and some just misunderstood. The deluded, the depressed, the alcoholic, the epileptic, the head-injured, the backward and the psychopathic were, like a potpourri of problems, mixed together and sent 'up the hill'. Indeed, the classification of mental illness was crude for much of the nineteenth and early twentieth century.

On the other side of the world, in Germany, a brilliant psychiatrist Emil Kraepelin wrote a mental health masterpiece that became the bedrock of modern psychiatric classification. The English translation of Kraepelin's work was published in two volumes, the first in 1919 and the second in 1921. In the second volume of his magnum opus he delineated from the morass of madness a specific mental illness called 'manic-depressive insanity'. It is also called manic-depressive illness, or just simply manic depression. Although the old term manic depression is still occasionally used, in the 21st century it goes by the modern label 'bipolar disorder'. And it remains an extraordinary and intriguing illness. Most people have some vague idea of how bipolar disorder expresses itself—that is, a mental illness where people have 'highs' and 'lows'. For our story, its description is crucial, so we need to know more about manic depression. Typically, manic depression begins in late adolescence or early adulthood—at the prime of life. And it runs in isolated attacks: sometimes the person suffers from mania, at another time, depression. It is an illness that has some remarkable features. One of these is that between episodes of illness, that is, between episodes of mania and depression, a person can remain perfectly well, as well and as normal as the most sane person on earth. And they can remain well in between episodes for years at a time.

When a sufferer becomes manic, the essential features are an exaltation of mood, rapid and pressured speech, delusions of wealth and grandeur, excitability, often expansive ideas to change the world, and an increased sexual drive. In the most profound states of mania the body and mind are completely lost to delusional excitement. The original descriptions by Kraepelin, taken from the late nineteenth and early twentieth century, remain unsurpassed:

> His surroundings appear to the patient to be changed; he sees
> St Augustine, Joseph with the shepherd's crook . . . God, the
> Virgin Mary. Statues salute him by nodding; the moon falls
> down from the sky; the trumpets of the day of judgment are
> sounding. He hears the voice of Jesus, speaks with God and

the poor souls, is called by God dear son. There are voices in his ears; the creaking of the floor, the sound of the bells take on the form of words. The patient has telepathic connection with an aristocratic fiancée, feels the electric current in the walls, feels himself hypnotised; transference of thought takes place . . .

He cannot be silent for long; he talks and screams in a loud voice, makes a noise, bellows, howls, whistles, is over-hasty in speech, strings together disconnected sentences, words, syllables, mixes up different languages, preaches with solemn intonation and passionate gestures, abruptly falling from high-sounding bombast to humorous homeliness, threats, whining, and obscenity, or suddenly coming to an end in unrestrained laughter . . .

The patients make all sorts of plans, wish to train as singers, to write a comedy . . . they start senseless businesses, buy houses, clothes, hats, give large orders, make debts; they wish to set up an observatory, to go to America . . . kiss strange ladies on the streets, frequent public houses, commit all possible acts of debauchery . . . While they appear in company as jovial fellows, give large tips, stand treat, they quarrel with their superiors, neglect their duty, give up their situations for trifling causes, leave public-houses without paying.

Of course it takes little imagination to translate the above escapades into the modern day. Instead of a nineteenth-century public house, think of a manic patient in an RSL club playing poker machines until all their money is exhausted; or emptying a credit card in a single night in a casino; or putting a down-payment on a fifty-million-dollar waterfront property in Sydney; or setting up an on-line business to sell secret cures for the problem of global warming; or placing a deposit on a third Porsche; or betting over the internet from one's bed 24 hours a day; or slapping on a GoPro helmet to film oneself jumping from a third-storey apartment, believing one can fly; or driving 160 kilometres per hour in a suburban street; or communicating with NASA to control the orbit of the planets. This is manic behaviour in the 21st century.

Such manic behaviour might last days or weeks or months. And in some cases, especially in the early twentieth century when there was no treatment, it could last as long as several years. Invariably these manic patients were admitted to asylums like Beechworth. Then, over time, if they managed to survive, the mania burnt itself out, and the person might become perfectly normal, waking from this furious delirium. When they looked about them, they had done great destruction to themselves and their families.

Sometimes patients remained well for months, even years. But almost inevitably another episode would grip them. Sometimes this was another manic episode, but it was just as likely to be an episode of depression.

In this deep and stagnant melancholia, thoughts slowed into viscous dribbles, barely budging, and a mood could plummet into the most profound state of despair; for most of us, the despair is not imaginable.

It is to Kraepelin again we turn and a snippet this time will do, because his description is almost unbearable to read to its end:

> The torment of the states of depression . . . engenders almost in all, at least from time to time, weariness of life, only too frequently also a great desire to put an end to life at any price . . . The patients, therefore, often try to starve themselves, to hang themselves, to cut their arteries; they beg that they may be burned, buried alive, driven out into the woods and there allowed to die.

Early death was common in untreated manic depression, suicide rates high.

Lives were lived out in this never-ending cycle of reckless exaltation and miserable lows. Patients might have dozens of admissions to asylums.

In 1936 the cause of manic depression was utterly mysterious. Some held that there might be a physical disorder ticking away in the body that brought it on; others assumed that something in the person's upbringing was at fault. Whatever one's belief, it remained the case that little could be done to treat it. Indeed, in the whole of psychiatry, there was not a single medication that specifically treated any mental illness. Of course there were pills and potions, like a mad-hatter's apothecary, which sometimes soothed, even knocked out patients for a while. But when patients woke from this drugged slumber they awoke as mad as before. The only ally doctors and nurses had was time.

4

During his time at Beechworth, John kept up a steady stream of letters to Jean in Melbourne. At first, the formality of the era overwhelmed intimacy and he started letters with a prim 'Dear Nurse Charles', written with all the passion of a job application; but in no time the stiffness was overthrown by romantic desires. Soon his letters were addressed to his 'Dear Jinnie'. In early 1937 John left Beechworth and returned to Melbourne; he and Jean made a decision to marry.

John and Jean were wed on 1 November 1937 at Melbourne's premier Catholic cathedral, St Patrick's. Family oral history has it that John had little money for an engagement ring and was too poor to invite guests. Instead, their meagre reception took place at the house his parents occupied on the grounds of Mont Park Hospital for the Insane, not, we imagine, the venue his bride might have envisioned when agreeing to a betrothal. Just a single photo exists of this reception, but in brilliant sunshine it captures a post-nuptial moment of bliss as John wraps a loving arm around the waist of his new bride. That they are on the grounds of a hospital for the insane seems inconsequential to them both.

The next phase of the story, it seems, has been repeated many times over the generations; children and grandchildren are able to recite the events at will. After his near-death from pneumonia, John had ditched his fashionable motorbike and purchased a Dodge coupé. The car was one of those flashy American jobs with exquisite maroon upholstery and the capacity to be a sporty two-seater. Jean and John tossed their few worldly possessions into the boot of the car, put the hood down and roared eastward out of Melbourne to Lakes Entrance, where they stayed at the evocatively named Robin Hood Inn, and then motored up the eastern seaboard of Australia to Sydney. And from there, as their honeymoon ended, they drove directly to Beechworth Asylum where a fully furnished doctor's cottage awaited them.

John and Jean took walks every evening on the asylum grounds at Beechworth; he loved nature and observed with an unhurried eye each unfolding flower and, in the gloaming, listened for the receding calls of birdlife as night fell. Jean fondly remembered 'he always looked at the skies; and he adored the magpies'. John seemed more relaxed this time round at Beechworth, taking an active part in patient activities. The patients held a monthly dance and in a rush of egalitarianism John waltzed with his patients. It was a time when embracing a patient while doing the rumba was deemed normal, even 'therapeutic', if dancing can be reduced to such a dull clinical term. And it forged a humanising link between doctor and patient that seems forever lost.

For some time John was the lone doctor at Beechworth and, indeed, when the hospital chemist fell ill John was required to stir and mix and prepare his own prescriptions. It was a chemical artistry he seemed to take to. But of all the events that occurred during this time at Beechworth, one remains foremost, and it came about when an observant attendant noticed a peculiar bruise in a male patient as the patient prepared to take a shower.

Asylums were segregated strictly along gender lines. Half of the hospital was male; the other half female. The shower parade in the morning was an asylum ritual. Attendants would shout at patients to rise from their beds and take a shower. In this belligerent and blunt world, Christian names were dropped, beds were rattled and patients prodded to get going of a morning. Stripped naked, patients were herded together, and goaded towards a communal shower. The line shuffled forward, naked flesh visible to the attendants, who could look for any signs of disease such as a rash or head lice. On one particular morning, an attendant noted bruising at first in one patient, and then in several others. The attendant drew this observation to John's attention.

John scrutinised, with a purposeful gaze, these blood-crimson welts on the skin of several men. The obvious and immediate conclusion he came to, or at least feared, was violence at the hands of some thuggish attendant. He returned to his cottage, Jean recalling his puzzlement: 'I must find out if they have been injured by the attendants or given a belting.' John examined, in his inquisitive way, all possible solutions. As he thought back to how his fingers gingerly pressed the soft flesh of these men, he rose to the occasion and another suggestion came to him: 'Maybe it is a lack of [nutritious] food.' It turned out to be an inspired hunch.

Jean remembers the appalling food prepared for patients, cooked in 'great big boilers, huge boilers until everything tasted the same. I mean you couldn't tell stewed pears from meat or from vegetables.' John, experimentally minded, set about proving his suspicion that it was a lack of nutrients that led to the bruising. His methodical work revealed a lack of vitamin C in the food; the patients at Beechworth had scurvy. Scurvy, the dreaded disease of early mariners on the high seas—a disease of bloated flesh and swollen joints, loose teeth and soft bleeding gums—had taken root in asylums. John wrote to his father in Melbourne. Word spread quickly. This discovery was a gloriously symphonic moment in a young doctor's life, and a turning point in the care of the mentally ill in Australia. Within a short time, the first dietician to be appointed in a Victorian mental hospital commenced work at Mont Park.

Not long after this, John and Jean returned to Melbourne and took up accommodation in the small asylum at Bundoora for returned servicemen, just over the road from Mont Park Hospital.

———

Two events marked the year of 1938 for John. The first, and most important, was the birth of John and Jean's first child, Jack, on 25 October.

When Jean married, in line with the expectations of the era, her nursing career ended overnight. Whether she harboured ambitions to continue as a nurse we don't know. But clearly this young woman who came second in her state nursing examinations was someone of fine intelligence. From the start of married life, Jean saw herself, as did everyone else, as an organised and capable homemaker.

The second event in 1938 was John's completion of an MD, or 'Doctor of Medicine', a postgraduate degree in medicine. This extra study was not expected of a medical doctor but, if nothing else, it reflected an inner ambition to be a scientific psychiatrist. When Jean questioned the value of yet more study and whether this was common, John retorted: 'Not in my department. But I still want it. You're a better doctor if you've done this.'

As part of his postgraduate study John was required to dissect a human brain. So a wet human brain stored in a chamber pot found its way into the Cade household. A freshly cut brain sloshing about on her dining room table was not part of Jean's notion of a newlywed's household but, in negotiations that would become commonplace, John got his way. The brain and the lingering smell of its pungent preservative was a vivid memory Jean could easily recall 50 years after the event. When Jean's girlfriends got wind of her engagement to a doctor studying psychiatry, they sniggered behind raised hands. 'All my friends said to me', whispered Jean as if talking about a murder, '"You're going to marry a psychiatrist in a mental hospital!" and I would say with a superior attitude with my nose in the air, "Only for a little while and then he's going into private practice".'

Secretly Jean was irritated with John's lack of interest in private work, social respectability and the capacity to earn more money. Jean overheard the smirking wives of private psychiatrists talk snidely of doctors like John 'as the poor little slum boys; they had no money; no one knew them; they had no name', whereas their own husbands were all in plush private practices in Collins Street. Sixty years later, in the late 1990s, Jean could still mimic the superior-sounding socialites of Melbourne she endured in her early married life. With a high-pitched mocking affectation and nose raised to the ceiling, she crowed: 'Oooooh! You're married to a loony-bin doctor!'

The private psychiatrists might have seen themselves as the cream of society but to John, they curdled before his eyes. More than ever, he was determined to remain a doctor who worked inside an asylum, attracted by 'the unrivalled opportunities' and 'the wealth of clinical material' in mental hospitals to study mental illness

In April 1939, John became a founding member of an association of Victorian mental hospital doctors dedicated to doing experimental studies to improve the lot of patients. Between July 1939 and September 1940 he was extremely productive, generating two research publications outside his usual work. One of them broke new ground in Australia, involving an unlikely pairing between a mental hospital doctor, and two noted medical researchers. One of John's partners was Frank Macfarlane Burnet, later to win a Nobel Prize in Medicine; another was Dora Lush, who was to die tragically during the Second World War as a result of a laboratory accident.

Events overtook any aspiration of John's to undertake further medical research. On 3 September 1939, Australia's Prime Minister, Robert Menzies, had declared that the nation was at war with Germany.

John was just a few weeks short of his 28th birthday when he enlisted. Filial duty was partly to blame. While a medical

student, 'My father, a pillar of Empire . . . had urged me to join
the Melbourne University Rifles and . . . I dutifully agreed.' But to
enlist in the army and leave Australia was altogether more difficult. John was torn. 'I didn't want to be dragged into it.' Having
been a member of the Citizen Military Forces for several years, one
evening 'we were summoned, to stand strictly to attention' when
John and his unit were 'berated . . . for our laggard cowardice in
not joining the AIF', the Australian Imperial Force:

> We were dumbfounded. The PM had told us not to be in a hurry.
> Australia was in no danger (this was Pig Iron Bob), remember,
> who was flogging Australian iron ore to the Nips, who slung it
> back at us less than two years later. So incensed were we by this
> tirade that we joined the AIF *en masse* only a few days later.
>
> I had to go down to the Caulfield Racecourse reception
> centre. There was a tall, handsome young man immediately
> in front of me in the queue of recruits, sporting a toothbrush
> moustache. I could not have known that he was [Dr] John Park,
> an Empire Games sprinter . . .

It was the first time John had clapped eyes on Dr John Park. They
were to become the closest of friends during their time in the army.

Several days later, Captain John Cade, now fully measured-up for
his uniform, prepared Jean for the lengthy aliquots of time he would
be away from home—training at the army camps near Seymour, at
Torquay and at Bonegilla near Albury. In mid-July, when the 8th
Division of the AIF formed, John commenced full-time with the Army.

Meanwhile, heavily pregnant, Jean set about scouring suburban
Melbourne for a family home. When on leave from the army, John—
in his freshly pressed army uniform—came to inspect her choices.
In the end, they settled on the middle-class suburban enclave of
Eaglemont, house number 38, in a street called The Righi. John
and Jean's second child, David, was born on 14 August 1940, and
The Righi would be home to Jean and her two boys while John
was overseas.

John's life was about to unfold in an uncannily similar way to his father's. And so, like the military reprise it was, John showed the world that he was no 'coward' and made final preparations to fight for his country.

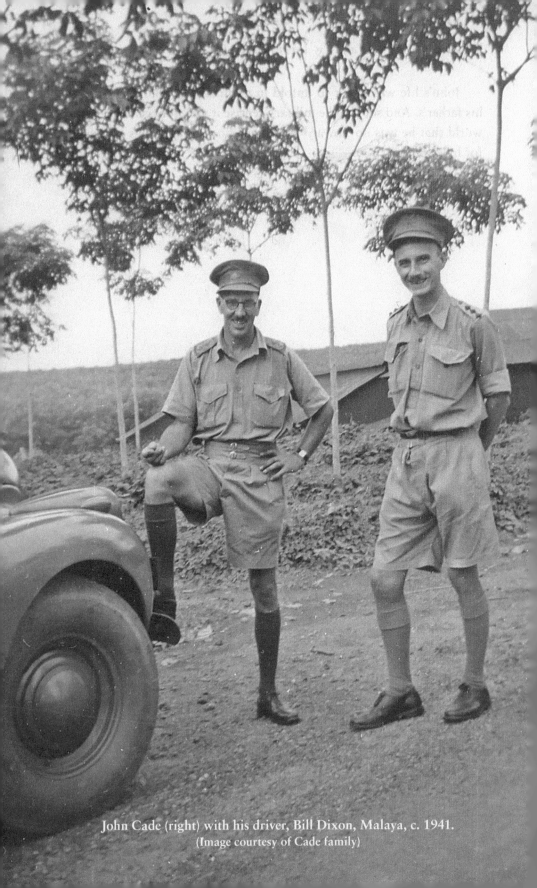

John Cade (right) with his driver, Bill Dixon, Malaya, c. 1941.
(Image courtesy of Cade family)

PART 2

The
Interminable
Years

JOHN CADE: *The war years*

I was never posted as a psychiatrist. Any psychiatric duties were incidental to my general regimental medical responsibilities as the senior company commander in a Field Ambulance . . . For some reason—I hope it was because of my specialist inclinations—I early attracted the nickname of the 'mad major'.

...he question of scrap iron for Japan, right away h...
...I was going to be done with it.

...that this Indonesian bid for independence is only...
...read dissatisfaction by the peoples of the East wi...
...ver lordship. The same problem is demanding solu...
...Burma and Indo China...

...of political speculation. Regarding leave, alo...
...ut at 28 days immediately following disembar...
...k or so in a convalescent camp (probably at Bel...
...l over haul, followed by another 30 days leave...
...are not sure of yet is whether we will get i...
...cumulated recreation leave which would amo...
...70-80 days. I suppose the department will...
...me as soon as possible - well, they will have...
...and I, darling, are entitled to a pretty good...
...that, I feel so rusty medically, that I simp...
...if possible three months post-graduate stud...
...like to do a month at St Vincents, a month at...
...a fortnight at the Eye and Ear, leaving a mo...
...swinging - all provided we can keep the depar...
...then to work - as you guessed in one of your e...
...old brain box is simmering with ideas. I be...
...riod of waiting has allowed many of my no...
...try to crystallise, and I'm just bursting to p...
...test. If they work out, they would represent a...
...the knowledge of...

5

Captain John Cade said his final lingering goodbyes to Jean and his two small boys just outside The Righi. 'Little did I think it would be five long years before I ever saw them again.'

Jack Cade was not yet three years old when his father left for war, David nearly six months. Today, Jack can take you back to the exact spot where he stood over 70 years ago watching his father leave. 'It was right on this spot,' he said, pointing to the driveway just outside the front gate. 'Mum was there, holding David in her arms.' From the driveway it is easy to sweep an eye along the sleepy suburban street, up a gentle incline and past the line of Federation-style houses; little has changed in over seven decades. Jack easily recaptures the vision of his uniformed father, neat and trim, striding along the footpath, lugging a suitcase, steadily ascending the slope of the street, not looking back at his wife and boys. With David in the crook of her arms, Jean peered up the street at her disappearing husband. Jack recalls his father's khaki shape getting smaller and smaller, until his dad looked no more than a toy soldier. At the top of the street, in a blink, his father turned left and was gone.

Jack remembers all this from his childhood. No doubt his memory has been embroidered over time; but if emotion counts for something, and surely it must, that moment of departure in 1941 was relived as if it were yesterday.

When John arrived at Bonegilla army camp, just outside Albury, he found it 'all bustle and preparation'. The younger recruits about him glowed with the anticipation of pulling out, 'thrilled when the day arrived for us to leave camp'; an older John was more circumspect, and wrote to Jean whenever time allowed. When the time came to depart, John boarded the train with the rest of the 2/9th Field Ambulance—all impelled by their unifying belief in the need to protect Australia—and set forth for Sydney. The old rattler rocked and swayed its way through southern New South Wales, John remembering: 'It was a miserable night journey packed as we were like sardines in ancient "dog-box" carriages.' Threading through the outer suburbs of Sydney, the train slowed and slid like a serpent between houses, 'the waving and cat-calls and long festoons of a certain essential toilet commodity trailing along the outside of the carriages . . .' The groggy garrison finally pulled in at Darling Harbour and left behind their toilet-papered carriages; in no time they found themselves on a ferry in Sydney Harbour, cutting through the waves towards the *Queen Mary*, berthed and camouflaged just outside Taronga Park Zoo.

John stepped aboard the *Queen Mary*—a floating palace for the decadent in peacetime, now refitted as the world's largest troop transport ship—and stood agog at its array of bronze statues and 'Hollywoodian' opulence. And then, in stiff competition with the officers streaming on board, he nabbed a first-class cabin. With typical Cade curiosity he studied a bidet, walking around it to better understand its function.

One of John's first written observations on board is unexpectedly acerbic. 'The stewards were enormously fat great Poms who could hardly pass each other in the corridors.' And, when informed that the plump 'Poms' were a wealthy duo who 'owned a row of houses in Plymouth', he digs his dagger in deeper. 'They were never tipped either.'

As the *Queen Mary* prepared to leave the harbour, the governor-general, came aboard with full pomp and wished the 6000 men well; a military band played and John, always the quietest of men, silently looked about him. His two brothers—Frank and David—were on other ships in this convoy, heading elsewhere to battle. The *Queen Mary* raised anchor and pulled out of Sydney Harbour on 4 February, their destination still unknown to most of the men on board. Along with her, a trifecta of accompanying ships—the *Mauretania*, the *Nieuw Amsterdam* and the *Aquitania*—sailed to war.

Soon after leaving the port of Fremantle, the convoy's first stop, the *Queen Mary* peeled away from the remaining ships, which were headed for the Middle East, and, in a lumbering arc, rounded the rear of the other vessels and powered her way towards Singapore. The last memory John had of this moment was of listening to the trumpeting calls and fading cheers of the men on board the remaining three ships as the *Queen Mary* churned her way northwards.

Life on board the palatial *Queen Mary* was rather bizarre for a warship—deck games during the day, dancing at night. Dr John Park, now the closest of friends with John, and eye-catchingly handsome, was a beacon for the heavily outnumbered female nurses. John Cade mischievously wrote to Jean about John Park and his amorous endeavours:

> Great goings-on tonight. There is a dance and the competition promises to be extraordinarily keen as there are about fifty nurses and twelve times that number of officers. It's amusing to watch the jockeying for positions. Our glamour boy has been putting in some good spade work all day and we are watching the fruit of his labours with the greatest of interest.

As tropical waters were entered, John caught sight of flying fish; within minutes the national pastime of a casual wager was underway. Men crowded towards the ship's railings, eagerly taking odds and laying down cash on how far the next fish could fling itself out of the waves. Meanwhile, inside, John was required to give repeated and tedious medical lectures to the men. Later in life he groaned: 'I gave endless lectures on tropical medicine and venereal disease among the prostitutes of South East Asia. We issued condoms and mercury ointment. The padres preached. The commanding officers commanded. Result nil.' At least that was the consequence of all that lecturing and preaching once the men hit shore and the sniff of sex was in the air.

———

The *Queen Mary* docked at the wharfs of Singapore on 18 February. At the water's edge, stick-legged vendors surrounded the men, the piquant aromas from their spiced foods foreign to Australian nostrils. These new scents soon mixed with the heavy air of wet and decay from the 'stinking hot and humid' jungle, nearly overwhelming the Australians. By now John's once-fresh uniform stuck to him like a leech and he had to peel away the moist clothing that sucked on his skin; although constantly wet, he never felt clean. Clad in Bombay Bloomers, the men wandered the streets before taking a train from Singapore to Malaya. The northwards-bound train chugged 'through the jungle most of the night, most of us sleepless and standing and savouring the strange smells of the tropics' before arriving at their destination, Port Dickson, on the western edge of the Malay Peninsula. Weary and dripping wet, they stepped from the train at 3 am, and marched to their barracks five kilometres away, arriving before dawn and, as John wrote, 'thankfully threw down our gear to collapse on the hard concrete floors for an hour or two . . .'

John acclimatised as best he could to the tropics, preparing his men for the inevitable injuries and illnesses of war. There remains a wonderful photograph from this time of anticipation. It shows John kitted out in full khaki uniform—short-sleeved shirt and knee-length shorts—standing on the deck of an open timber verandah. It is a steamy tropical day and his clothes are drenched with sweat.

John's admiring eyes are fixed on his great friend, Dr John Park, who stands a few metres away—lithe and athletic—ready to attack an imaginary Japanese soldier. John Park brandishes a bayonet, dealing death to his imagined foe. With his pencil-thin moustache and twinkling eyes, Park is a dead ringer for Errol Flynn, and grinning like a buccaneer on the high seas, he is just about ready to skewer the villain and whisk away the girl.

Once in Malaya it didn't take long for the ill and injured to accumulate. Men, unused to the tropics, quickly succumbed to fungal infections. 'Infection of the crutch and scrotum areas was known as dhobi itch . . . nasty dull red itchy rash with a slightly raised edge spreading steadily outwards' and tinea of the feet crippled soldiers; and then, of course, there was 'VD, the curse of all armies'.

One of John's roles as an officer was to weed out the unfit for war, even at this late stage of proceedings. Sometimes this was for physical reasons, sometimes psychological, occasionally moral. John was a compassionate man, but as much as he supported the underdog and the ill, he detested the spineless:

> Before the outbreak of hostilities we repatriated a considerable number of men . . . who could not stand up to tropical conditions—. . . dermatitis or asthenia . . . neurotic reactions of various kinds and plain cold feet. So we had time for a ruthless pruning process of the unfit and the unwilling, in whatever guise the unwillingness manifested itself. There is no end to human ingenuity when the reward is a return ticket home.

It was the strangest of times in Malaya—preparing for war but not quite sure when it would arrive. To amuse themselves the 2/9th Field Ambulance formed its own Australian Rules football team. Its captain was 21-year-old Harold Ball, who had recently held the 1940 Grand Final Cup aloft as a member of the victorious Melbourne Football Club. Ball was possessed of a big head and square jaw; it was a mug that said 'footballer' even before you knew he was one, and at six foot two Harold Ball was a quelling sight.

John was promoted to major prior to the 2/9th moving to Mersing, a town on the eastern seaboard of the Malay Peninsula. We have one telling memory of him from about this time. John never spoke about this event, or at least never took the time to write about it, but fortunately for us, Jack Sammons, a member of the 2/9th did. It is transcribed in Carl Johnson's mammoth book on the 8th Division, Australian Army Medical Corps, *Carrying On*.

As Jack Sammons described the incident:

A dispatch rider was coming in from Mersing and he and his bike parted company. The result was a very badly cut and scratched soldier, who had lost a lot of blood and was urgently in need of a transfusion. A doctor, on loan to us from a British unit, was an orderly medical officer on duty and called for blood donor volunteers. Paul Payne's blood was comparable and he reported to make his donation. Our visiting medical officer botched the job and was splattering Paul's blood all around the aid post when Major John Cade—our company commander and a doctor—arrived on the scene. He was ropeable and made serious threats, which, if he carried them out; would have had very disastrous consequences—especially as it was one doctor against another. Fortunately, things quietened down. John took over and nothing more was to come out of what looked like an international incident.

John's keen eye observed how the army cooks tossed out so much refuse; and that it was being collected by an old, bent Malayan man and his grandson. Within months John wrote that the boy, by just eating these food scraps with a few bits of enrichment tossed in by the cooks, grew rapidly into a robust boy. John marvelled at this change in human constitution in a growing boy and later in life reflected: 'I have never forgotten this lesson in nutrition.'

He writes home to Jean of what he observes in Malaya: of luscious pawpaw, of scorpions larger than dinner plates and king cobras the length of a bus. A pet python of one soldier drapes about the men at 16 feet in length and sleeps at night in the man's locker; a colony of chattering monkeys entertain him; a 14-year-old boy from Australia has somehow snuck into the ranks of the men; mosquitoes are their enemy and everyone fears malaria. After he drives through the kampongs of Malaya he writes at length about the dozens of curious children running to him; of the 'nondescript hens and chickens, bantam roosters, numerous goats of all sizes . . . There are not many dogs and what there are [are] mangy looking mongrels.' He wryly observes a meditating yogi sitting on nails, and as an aside wonders (pragmatically) how and when he gets up to go to the toilet; John bangs his boots every morning for spiders and watches a column of ferocious marching tropical ants: he is consumed by the sights and smells of Malaya. Of his two small boys in suburban Melbourne he writes: 'I hope neither of them will have grown up too much before Daddy returns, because he's missing such a lot.' All the while John waits for the Japanese to attack.

On 8 December 1941, the waiting was over; before dawn the Japanese landed on the beach near Kota Bharu on the Malay Peninsula. John and the 2/9th—safe for the moment—were well to the south of the invading Japanese. But in the distance a storm brewed; not thunder, but the distant rumble of exploding shells. The jungle was restless; thousands of Japanese foot-soldiers, like the marching ants John had observed, coiled their way south. The Japanese streamed down the narrow Malay Peninsula and attacked with unfettered ferocity, meeting with spasmodic and uncoordinated resistance from the Allied troops. The Allied strategic plans, it turned out, were abysmal and chaotic; the required thinking had not been done and resources were inadequate. The Allied forces took flight and fled southwards; a shambling mess of soldiers and displaced civilians—hungry and beaten—drained towards the island of Singapore. It was clear that the British were unable to offer the protection so many Australians back home had hoped for, even expected. By the end of January 1942 this river of refugees had withdrawn to Singapore, still regarded as an impregnable fortress by many, and here they hoped to stage a final battle.

6

Jean often sat at her Singer treadle sewing machine, stitching new clothes and costumes for the boys, her right foot rhythmically rising and falling.

David fondly remembered:

> Mum made a lot of our clothes during the war. She stitched
> suits for Jack and me; for Cowboys and Indians. She made the
> Indian suits out of sugar bags, which she dyed dark brown then
> hemmed them; and she made headbands. We had chooks and
> used blue-coloured feathers from the chooks and roosters in the
> headbands. And we had a vest each, with a sheriff's badge on it.
> And she made wooden swords.

While John was at war, Jean lived by the rigid rationing rules of the time. Everything was carefully counted out, measured and marked; nothing wasted, whether food or clothing—her two chief preoccupations in caring for Jack and David. Before he left for war, John had excavated a huge vegetable garden out the back; Jean and the boys assiduously tended this to grow the greens the trio needed. With few cars on the road and even less petrol available, visitors were rare at The Righi, and the Cades only occasionally ventured beyond their own suburb. Jean's next-door neighbour Yvonne, in an effort

47

to lessen the isolation, cut a gate through the fence separating their backyards.

Jean still had the gorgeous Dodge coupé. But on a meagre ration of 4 gallons a month, driving was a luxury she indulged sparingly. Her mother-in-law, Ellen, insisted (4 gallons or not) that Jean and the boys come to visit her and John's father who, although he had officially retired in 1940, was intermittently filling in as acting medical superintendent at Mont Park Mental Hospital. So most Sundays Jean packed the two neatly attired boys into the Dodge and drove about 15 minutes to their destination. The boys remember the car as a beauty with 'a seat that shot up in the back', to make it a two-seater. The round trip just about exhausted the petrol quota. To Jack and David it was a touch of exotica to drive northwards from The Righi and out of the depths of suburbia to where there were 'no houses, only paddocks full of Scotch Thistles', until this trio of Cades arrived at the elaborate wrought iron gates that marked the grand entrance to the asylum. Mont Park was built with splendour in mind, and John's father—when in charge—lived in the gracious two-storey superintendent's house. Once out of the car the boys larked about in the grounds. Most of all they remember games around an Aboriginal canoe tree, 'a big old gum'. When summoned into the superintendent's house, they sat somewhat sullenly 'in a dingy parlour with a coal fire' until released to play. Best of all, though, was the afternoon tea prepared by Amy, the mental-hospital patient who acted as the housemaid for the superintendent. Amy's speciality for these Sunday afternoon wartime visits, and the boys' favourite, was to roll out a varnished trolley, on top of which sat a batch of fresh scones, jam and tea.

Back at The Righi, some of these wartime moments at home are frozen in three black and white photographs. In one photograph, taken on a particularly sunny Melbourne day, Jack sits in a toy motor car that he can propel with his feet and steer around the yard; nearby, David sits on a tricycle shaped like a horse's head.

The two boys, sweet and innocent, look deeply into the lens of the camera. In another photograph, Jean sits with the boys in the yard: an impish-looking Jack and the blond curls of David steal the scene; Jean, for her part, seems preoccupied with faraway thoughts. In another, Jack and David are immaculately dressed for the camera in shorts and shirts, their hair impeccably swept to the side, not a strand out of place. Jean is a picture-perfect, young lipsticked woman with a string of pearls and a prim knee-length skirt; she strikes a pose that is motherly and doting. These warm and innocent days inoculated the boys from the war. Their radiant world was defined by the shelter of the house and the warmth of its garden. The unthreatening front- and backyards of The Righi offered them a secure world; nothing dangerous here, unless it was the antics of the boys:

> We had a red racing car. A peddle car with a steering wheel. Our driveway was steep to the garage. Jack and I would get to the top of the driveway and take it in turns to hurtle down as fast as we could, heading straight to the garage. At the last second we had to swerve and miss the garage and head around the corner into the backyard. Mum, I'm sure, thought we'd kill ourselves.

The boys played out these days in a world of fantasy, of heroes and villains, where Indians fought cowboys and everyone came in for lunch—and then they'd fight again all afternoon. The tranquillity of suburban Melbourne belied a world breaking apart. The real war beyond their front fence was not something the boys really understood. Even now, seen through the sometimes vivid, sometimes hazy aperture of childhood memories, Jack and David recall with immense happiness this blissful backyard life.

7

As the Japanese swarmed down the Malay Peninsula, John and the 2/9th Field Ambulance, along with all the Australian and Allied troops, retreated. The troops drained towards the southern tip of the Malay Peninsula where, over a narrow stretch of ocean, the island of Singapore—a tiny plot of land only 50 kilometres long and 26 kilometres wide—awaited them. By the beginning of February 1942, tens of thousands of Allied troops crammed into this tiny island. It would be their final refuge.

John Cade and the 2/9th were holed up in its northwest corner helping to ferry and treat the wounded. Frantically, he and his men stemmed bleeding, splinted broken bones, dug trenches and erected tents. Injured Australians kept pouring in from Malaya across the Johore Strait into Singapore. Then the Japanese bombing began. Swarms of buzzing bombers, engines rumbling like a hive of agitated bees, dropped their whistling bombs from the heavens to blister the earth below.

John recalled:

I had a little tent at our Main Dressing Station in a rubber plantation on northwest Singapore Island. The enemy shelling became heavier and heavier as their invasion hourly approached. As I lay down one night exhausted I covered my head with my tin hat. Then I shifted it to my chest. Finally, convulsively I shoved it over my genitals. Such were the varying orders of priority.

Another time at this same location, as a result of an air-raid warning, I had shepherded all wounded and sick into slit trenches and then as I was making my way back to HQ dugout found myself caught in the open by the scream of falling bombs. I burrowed into what I fondly imagined was a slight saucer shaped depression in the ground, face down; then thought, 'No, I'd like to see what's coming' and turned face up.

John remained for some time in that position, on his back, face up and limbs unmoving, mesmerised by the insanity of the moment. As he peered into the sky the bombs continued to fall: it seemed impossible one would not hit. It was not the only time in those fateful weeks that John expected to die.

The great fear of all ambulance men was to leave behind a wounded soldier to the caprice of the advancing Japanese; all effort and courage bent towards preventing this. It was in such a determined mood that John, in an ambulance, accidentally found himself behind enemy lines, surrounded by Japanese soldiers. John recalled the surreal and dangerous moment:

> I was on reconnaissance trying to locate X battalion, the 'odds and sods', not knowing that it had even then been wiped out to a man, to provide them with an RMO [Regimental Medical Officer] when my driver and I ran into an ambush in pitch dark (we didn't dare use head lights) and my reaction was (I was standing on the running boards—they had them in those days—directing my driver) terror, I hissed inside the car—'Reverse and turn and let's bugger off quick!' He did, thank God. The Nips weren't after such small fry as us . . .

This act of cool-headedness—evaluating the position rapidly and immediately dealing with it—became legendary within the 2/9th Field Ambulance. Over the years it has been recited and, without doubt, finessed to suit the mood of the occasion. Like all war stories, the light and shade varies in the telling, the mix of truth and fiction differing from person to person.

In the final frantic days before surrender, John was tearing about, caring for the injured in the city of Singapore, 'charging round the aisles of St Andrew's Cathedral'. To make way for the wounded, pews were pitched outside, stretchers and mattresses carted inside. John moved about the battle-wounded and dying on the floor of the cathedral; some lay still, bleeding, unable to move; others writhed in agony. The cathedral floor groaned with bodies of soldiers and civilians, though in dying there was little to distinguish between them. The fetid cathedral air was thick with the sounds of the wounded and the smell of dead flesh and soggy bandages wrapped around dying limbs. Decades afterwards, John could still remember the acrid blend of blood and faeces and smoke, a sticky scent that clung to his nostrils. Whatever reserves of energy John possessed he spent in 'slugging hundreds and hundreds of exhausted and panic-stricken troops' with sedatives 'from a huge syringe'. John, for the most part, was endowed with a capacity to curtain off his immediate reaction to these obscene images and do what was needed.

On 15 February the Allied command surrendered. Exhausted, John expected, along with all Allied prisoners, to be executed by the Japanese: 'The night of capitulation I expected to be my last. The Nip rough stuff were infiltrating the city centre and cutting down anything that moved.' Then, with the serenity of a man who believes his future is fixed, John fatalistically 'lay down on the grass beside [his] ambulance not expecting to survive the night'. When the following day dawned and he awoke still resting beside his ambulance, no one was more astonished than John that he was 'safe and sound'.

In the first anxious hours after surrender, John found himself in a post-apocalyptic city. George Aspinall, a fellow POW, secretly recorded a stunning series of grainy black and white photographs from this period after capitulation. The images show a city that has ceased to live. St Andrew's Cathedral, John's last refuge, appears eerily normal, a line of ready-to-use ambulances standing at attention; on the beaches, rocks are strewn about, like the disgorged remnants of a volcanic eruption. Among the rising spirals of smoke, three defeated men, more dead than alive, wander along the waterfront, lost. No Allied soldier had expected to surrender; they expected to fight and either win or lose. This was neither, and now they assembled in this netherworld, tens of thousands of numb soldiers, shuffling about, waiting for their Japanese conquerors to arrive.

As the triumphant Japanese swaggered into Singapore, the victors seemed dumbfounded by the problem at hand—what to do with over 50,000 captive Allied personnel and civilians? Their impromptu solution was to muster the tens of thousands and force them towards the southeast corner of the island, to a place called Changi. So, regardless of their state of health, wounded or otherwise, all soldiers were ordered to trudge the roughly 25 kilometres to Changi. John recalled with some considerable gratitude how, stretched out along the sides of the road, local residents, particularly the Chinese, extended their hands towards the Australian soldiers offering small kindnesses of bananas, water and coconuts.

It was several months after his incarceration as a prisoner of war that John found out that his closest friend—John Park—had been murdered in the mayhem as the Japanese attacked the island of Singapore. There are several versions of what happened but the following is about as close to the truth as anyone can get.

All was chaos and death in those final days as the Japanese invaded. A call came out to John Park that several Australian soldiers, wounded and without transport, were trapped and unable to retreat from the advancing enemy. Park and three other men gallantly responded: the first, a driver, was Harold Ball, the giant ruckman from the 2/9th Aussie Rules football team. After Ball there was another driver, William Lewis, and an orderly, Alf Woodman.

John Park and his three companions jumped into their ambulance, responding to the distress call 'without hesitation, consultation or loss of time' and drove into the haze of battle in the northwest corner of Singapore Island. They did not reappear.

Several months after the Allied surrender, Australian POW work parties were sent out by the Japanese to scour parts of the island for wood and the like. Surreptitiously they looked for dead Australian soldiers. They came across John Park.

Even when bodies were found like this, identifying them was made difficult by the accelerated decomposition in the hot atmosphere and constant rain. Looters, like vultures feeding upon carrion, often ransacked these Allied soldiers' bodies, and removed any valuables they could find. When Park was found, rumours flew around the camp about the grisly find and how the men died. One oral history handed down is that Park had been bound and then beheaded. The belief is that all the men were captured, tortured and executed, but what actually occurred is mired in uncertainty.

Park's death was a blow from which John never fully recovered. Jean just said her husband 'never got over that'. Even though he was a forgiving man, it seems likely that John never quite forgave the Japanese. One senses that John Cade felt he never was quite the man that Park was; not in an envious or grasping manner, but simply an acknowledgement that he had once had the privilege of knowing someone sublime. John wrote of Park that 'No one could know him and not love him', a tribute few could be accorded. Park was recommended for a posthumous Victoria Cross—but no award was ever bestowed.

_____

The name Changi referred to a large tract of land, a peninsula poking out from the eastern edge of Singapore Island. Its natural features were unprepossessing—low wooded sandy hills, marshes and mangrove swamp. Bounded by the ocean on three sides, it was the ideal location for a prison: no escape was possible via the sea and the fourth and final side was fenced with wire. Even this was somewhat tokenistic. If a desperate soldier made the decision to escape there was frankly nowhere to go and nowhere to hide. A white man was going nowhere in Southeast Asia.

After the war, Dr Michael Woodruff, a Changi POW, wrote:

> To keep us in place the Japanese initially drew a line on the map, and told us that any prisoner of war (POW) caught west of the line would be beheaded or shot; at the same time they offered a reward of five Japanese dollars to the locals for every prisoner they captured. This proved remarkably effective.

Within days over 50,000 men straggled into this prison ringed by water and wire. As they were leaving Singapore city and along the way, the soldiers opportunistically grabbed anything they thought might be of value during their imprisonment. They stuffed medicine into backpacks and loaded heavier equipment on to trucks; anything that could be pilfered or packed was brought along. Containers of Marmite and Vegemite—rich sources of B complex vitamins—were stashed into containers and hauled in. Knickknacks and entertainments of all kinds were conveyed: musical instruments, gramophone records, armfuls of books as well, tools of every description; anything in those frantic hours that was thought to be of value was nabbed, snatched or packed and taken.

Before the war, parts of Changi had been a staging point for British troops. So there were many relatively modern barrack buildings available for the troops to move into.

Bill Flowers, a private with the 2/9th Field Ambulance, described the location:

> It was a British secondment area where the British had quartered their soldiers before the war. There were many ground, first and second storey buildings ... It was ideal for the huge number of prisoners the Japanese had taken in Singapore. Of

course, when the British surrendered there were almost 40,000
British, almost 20,000 Australians . . . there was this huge
number. The Japanese wondered . . . what do we do with these
people? . . . Now, we settled into these buildings.

The Japanese, as puzzled as everyone else as to what might happen
next, allowed significant autonomy within the prison camp. As
a result, the prisoners were allowed to run their own show to a
large extent.

Almost immediately, tribal instinct took over, and the different
nationalities—primarily British, Australian and Dutch—adopted
separate areas, which they fenced and policed at the request of the
Japanese. Bill Flowers explained: 'In Changi, the different nationalities tended to stay together. You made mates with some UK, even
the Dutch blokes. But each area was relatively self-contained.' The
Australians largely took up a section called Selarang Barracks; the
British bunked down at Roberts Barracks. The barracks were close
to one another but the Australians and British largely kept to themselves although cooperation did take place.

There were six ring-locked areas in total. The one next to Roberts
Barracks was known as Roberts Hospital. It too was divided up into
a British wing of 2000 beds and an Australian wing catering for
1000 patients. In general, AIF patients were treated by Australian
doctors in Australian wards, and meticulous medical records were
kept. The latter was a key point of difference, as the British were lax
in medical record-keeping.

The pulse of Changi soon settled into a slow rhythm, the men
weighed down by heat and hunger. John remembered that it took
him about a week 'to recover from sheer exhaustion'. Most days
were drippy sorts of days; and every afternoon the tropical rains fell.
At 3 pm, just like a mid-afternoon cocktail at Raffles, the rain—on
schedule—came down. So intense was the humidity that even when
it stopped raining the wetness never entirely went away, leaving John

and his men feeling sticky and unwashed. At night, when all was quiet, the constant tap of water coming from somewhere ticked the night away.

This strange world was now John's home. Guards—some Korean, some Indian, some Japanese—all patrolled, but were sometimes not seen for days on end. In response a kind of laissez-faire market economy took root; some of the men took their chances by trading with the local population, bartering and bidding for what they could.

It was a world where men survived on their wits and scavenged their way through each day; inevitably pockets of ill-discipline flourished in darker corners. Many of the POWs entered Changi feeling betrayed by the ineptitude of their commanders and the uncertainty of the future vanquished the spirit of some. It was not long before dysphoria settled hard over the camp. As spirits sagged, a handful of soldiers turned to looting and pilfering; decency, along with truth, was an early casualty of war. The early dissolute and undisciplined behaviour of some troops needed to be curbed and was curbed. Discipline and routine among the Australian troops would be the long-term cornerstone of their survival. John later wrote that the most important psychiatric lesson he learned from Changi was 'the life saving value of high morale. As POW[s] we were internally superbly organized and disciplined with a continuation of the tough military hierarchical structure that we were used to ... It seemed ludicrous at the time, all this spit and polish and saluting among sick and starving men, but it was life saving.'

John settled into a medical routine, spending a good deal of time working in the hospital, looking after the men in his company. At times relations between the Australian and British hospital staff were tense. David Elder, a chief clerk with the Australians, penned these bitter and heartfelt lines many years afterwards: 'There was a very big difference between attitudes of the English and Australians regarding medical concerns. No Australian died without someone easing his passing. The British weren't like that.'

Difficulties between the two sectors in the hospital mattered more than was anticipated because, at its core, Changi was all about the care of wounded and sick men. All of a sudden, medical officers like John Cade were the most important men in the POW camp. It was the senior medical men, rather than the heads of fighting forces, who forwarded reports to the Japanese about inadequacies in food rations, drinking water, space for latrines, washing facilities and measures to control mosquito and fly breeding. By convincing the Japanese inspection teams that the camp would be decimated by disease without prompt action, senior doctors won major concessions.

We have snippets of memories of John from the men of the 2/9th Field Ambulance. All point to a quiet man, universally liked and with the gift of discretion; compassionate and stern and fair-minded in just the right mix. Decency was the fulcrum around which John based his POW life.

Survival in Changi revolved around food. Hunger eclipsed all else. Food is what everyone thought about, dreamt about. John, like everyone else, was preoccupied with 'the rations': 'We were relentlessly starved throughout and nutritional diseases . . . were universal. The food had to be rigorously rationed—weevilly rice, palm oil and stinking fish.' At times, in a semi-delirium, he fantasised about food, bountiful and ripe, and a future where he might sit at the table of 'luscious ravenous feasts'.

Rice was the universal food; disgust the universal response. In the early days of the systematic malnutrition foisted upon them by the Japanese, and before the Australian cooks knew how to cook and embellish it, rice was a gluggy mass plonked upon each POW's plate. George Aspinall's secretive series of photos captures one image of the men eating, sitting on their haunches, backs against a wall like a line of roosting pigeons, scooping the soggy rice from their plates into their mouths.

Unsurprisingly, vitamin deficiencies became apparent in the men from the very start. John suffered a debilitating 'attack of

Vitamin A deficiency' in the first three months of captivity and developed night blindness. Desperate for vitamin-rich food, as the shadows lengthened he slunk off into the twilight and traded his US Cyma wristwatch with local residents for a bag of raw peanuts and anything else that might supplement his diet. It was enough; his sight returned to normal.

All about, men fell sick with malaria, with diarrhoea, and with dysentery, John included. Vitamin B deficiencies were a scourge—the illnesses of beri-beri and pellagra prominent. Young men, without warning, collapsed and perished. A scratch in a weakened body unable to heal might lead to repulsive and deformed limbs, misshapen by spreading tropical ulcers. The hospital wards bulged. Even there, anything that could bite the men did so: bed bugs infested bunks at night, and scabies of the scrotum and penis led to uncontrollable scratching.

Nutrient deficiencies cut down even the strongest of the youths about John. And when brittle-boned boys dropped dead before his eyes, he slit them open at autopsy, quickly, before they putrefied under a tropical sun. It was a singular memory that revolted him in later life—not for the fact that he cut them open, because as a doctor this was expected of him, but because he was slicing into the bodies of severely malnourished boys. John Cade was not squeamish, but opening these young men up nearly broke him: 'All you found were great big fat livers and intestines that looked like sodden tissue paper.' John horrified himself when—mid-autopsy—he cracked a joke about lamb's fry for breakfast. Repulsed by his own insensitive words, he recoiled immediately. But it, nonetheless, tells us that in this cruel prison camp, even this most even-tempered of men could fantasise in the most twisted of ways.

———————

Although John was never posted as a psychiatrist, this being 'incidental to my general . . . medical responsibilities', within six months of captivity he was assigned to take 'care of the small 10–12 bed psychiatric ward in Changi plus the occasional consultation over the odd psychiatric case' in the general wards. As a result of this appointment, he soon attracted the affectionate moniker of the 'mad major'. The so-called Mental Ward that John ran was one of the few joint Australian–British wards in the hospital. That he was able to earn the respect of both forces, given the tensions between them, says a great deal about John's ability and diplomacy, especially given the suspicion psychiatry still attracted from some quarters. Psychiatrists in war, an unimpressed Winston Churchill suggested, could do the most damage of all to the morale of the fighting man:

> it would be sensible to restrict as much as possible the work of these gentlemen, who are capable of doing an immense amount of harm with what may very easily degenerate into charlatanry. The tightest hand should be kept over them and they should not be allowed to quarter themselves upon the Fighting services at the public expense. There are, no doubt, easily recognisable cases which may benefit from treatment of this kind, but it is very wrong to disturb large numbers of healthy, normal men and women by asking the kind of odd questions in which the psychiatrists specialise. There are quite enough hangers-on and camp followers already.

Churchill's view of psychiatry was hardly sophisticated, even if he had a rough-edged point to make. It is unlikely that John ever read Churchill's critique; he might have taken offence but it is unlikely. Because, like Churchill, John thought some psychiatry was an abominable mix of fanciful theories and little practical value. If he had ever met someone like John Cade, Churchill might have had cause to shift his hefty frame and view psychiatry from a more generous perspective.

The 'mental cases', as the psychiatrically unwell were unceremoniously dubbed, were first accommodated in a room on the ground floor of the Roberts Hospital. Matters stepped up when a British orderly, Private Morrison, 'was savagely attacked by a patient with a hatchet' and gravely injured, after which 'the Mental Cases were removed to a more commodious room' some distance away from the main body of patients. Presumably this increased everyone else's peace of mind, but it is a separation of care which continues to bedevil the treatment of the mentally ill to this day. A Private Nicholson who worked on the 'mental ward' remained wary:

> Eight at night to eight in the morning, twelve hour shifts. You sort of had to sit and face the ward ... and the row of beds each ... containing patients of varying degrees of insanity or mental condition ... You had to be very careful of what you stored; what could represent a weapon of some sort because they could use anything.

From the start there were men who were depressed and despondent. Suicide was reported to be rare, but John did note 'a few suicides of despair' early in captivity.

Occasionally a psychiatrically ill soldier might resist all efforts to be fed. Commanded by an unseen hand, he kept his mouth sealed and resisted any attempt to open it. Starvation, already at every soldier's door, was welcomed by these mentally damaged men—the depressed and the deluded—as a means to death.

Private Nicholson remembered lengthy attempts to get some of these soldiers to eat. The rigidly closed mouths of some had eventually to be prised open with a rough-hewn tool so they could be force-fed. And so, like a crowbar wedging open a locked window, the mouths of the mentally ill were jemmied open just enough for life-sustaining food to pour in.

Surrounded by the invalids of war—whether in the 'Mental Ward' or elsewhere—John's undeviating focus was on all the men in his care. He tended his fellow soldiers, coaxing life into broken bodies and sanity into mad minds. The truth is that this was a virtuoso performance by John and the other men who nursed and doctored these demoralised and disfigured men, done without any hint of applause. As malnourished soldiers in the general hospital piled up in their hundreds, John ploughed on. Ultimately, these men depended upon the quality of their medical care more than anything else in Changi. And sometimes it was just a thimbleful of care a man needed—a look or a touch—to hold on and live.

8

Changi was a world of constant tedium and occasional brutality. Bill Schmitt, an auctioneer in Adelaide before the war, tells of one such occasion when, for some unknown reason, he incurred the wrath of a Japanese guard:

Jap brutality . . . yeah, of course, they treated me bloody badly. Knocked me unconscious. I'd had malaria and then a bout of dysentery, one or the other, I can't remember which come first and I hadn't been out to work for a month or six weeks. Then I had to go to make up the numbers . . . I was shovelling the bloody sand and this Jap wasn't happy . . . I was so bloody weak and he grabbed me shoulder . . . and I don't know if I laughed at him or what but I did something that upset him and he bashed me. The next thing I know . . . I think he broke some ribs. He made a hell of a mess. Mouth and lips. Hit me with his fists 3 or 4 times and broke my nose.

This paroxysm of sadistic fury was not a commonplace act according to many POWs. For the most part, the men were left on their own by the guards. But not always.

In late August of 1942, the Japanese requested that all POWs sign a declaration not to attempt to escape from Changi. The Allied soldiers, in unison, refused to sign. As punishment, nearly 16,000 of them were ordered to mass in Selarang Square; they would be made to suffer beneath the Singapore sun until, spirits snapped, they signed the document.

A quota of the wounded and sick from the nearby Roberts Hospital also mustered in the square. Some patients were wheeled there on trolleys, some limped; others were carried. Many still bore injuries from bomb blasts or bullets; there were amputees with freshly hewn limbs recovering from surgery. Many were suffering from dysentery, malaria and vitamin deficiencies. This was absurdly cruel. It was not as if the prisoners were going anywhere. This was an act to visibly humiliate and crush the prisoners' spirit as much as any attempt to thwart escape from Changi.

As their circumstances grew more precarious, the thousands of men in the square neared breaking point. Still they refused to sign. On the third day, when the POWs apparent unpardonable act of refusal to sign persisted, the Japanese raised the stakes.

At about 4 pm, four men were summarily executed by firing squad on nearby Changi Beach. All four men—two Australians and two Englishmen—had previously tried to escape.

When news filtered back to the men in the square, it rippled in all directions like a whispered secret passed around a classroom. It was evident to everyone that there was little use in holding out. The miserable documents were signed by the troops, even though they held no weight—moral or material. For some time the stunned soldiers loitered a little before drifting to their barracks. The latrines and the refuse of 16,000 men were buried; soon all was normal again. To look at the tidied-up square several days later one would think nothing ever happened; certainly nothing criminally inhuman.

Somewhere in the midst of this barbaric farce John Cade was still, presumably, tending his patients. We know that when John reflected on this deeply repugnant moment, his hatred of the Japanese burned and left him 'under no illusions as to what our hosts were or were not capable of'.

When John looked at his worldly belongings they didn't amount to much. Years after the war he glowed with pride remembering how he'd kept his three precious razor blades sharp for years 'with the help of an old Marmite jar'. Tobacco, a rare pleasure for John, was hard to come by in Changi. The troops, inventive and entrepreneurial, concocted some smelly varieties known as 'Sikh's beard' and 'Granny's snatch'. John often scanned the ground for half-smoked cigarette butts, collecting them in the hollow of his cupped hands before mashing the titbits into a single smokeable fag. Jean disapproved of smoking, especially by pregnant women and by anyone inside a house, but in post-war years she took great pleasure in relaying some of John's POW stories. 'He was a big smoker, most of his life. He told me how they started tearing up and using Shakespeare and then the Bible.' John always knew when Red Cross parcels arrived in Changi: he saw the butts of American cigarette brands littered around the camp, and he knew the Japanese had ransacked and smoked the Red Cross packets for themselves.

At night John dreamed. He had many dreams in Changi. They were rarely sexual; it seems that there was little energy for them. Instead it was images of hatred that bulged in his brain at night: fantasising how he might escape, or, better still, humiliate and destroy his persecutors. All other thoughts, sex included, were sublimated into this: how to flee the enemy or destroy him. But preferably destroy. These were the droplets of acid that ate away at John as he slept.

By day he schemed to protect precious medicines from the Japanese. These medicines, especially morphine and antibiotics, were concealed about the camp. One such antibiotic was M&B 693, which was 'carefully hidden against Nip spot searches'. Years after the war, John's hardness towards his captors was still raw:

> The Nip and Korean guards were always getting the clap down
> in Lavender Street in Singapore Town and they were absolutely
> terrified of fronting up to their own MOs [Medical Officers]
> because the Nips had a very effective way of treating VD. You

were immediately shipped off to the front line. They knew we had M&B and they would come pleading for a bit but it was far too precious to let the little bastards have any.

———

Although John spent his entire three and a half years in Changi, many Allied soldiers didn't. The Japanese saw Changi as a repository of men, a storehouse of labour to supply an endless line of workers for the building of the Thai–Burma railway, and for brutal labour camps spread across an archipelago of islands from Borneo to Japan. From about the start of May 1942 the Japanese sent men to work on the Thai–Burma railway.

Lloyd Cahill was one of the men sent with 'F' force to work on the railway. Lloyd had just completed his intern year as a doctor at St Vincents Hospital in Sydney when he left Australia for the war. He met John Cade in Changi:

John, I knew him well. John was senior to me. He was a very good fellow. I regarded him as one of the best medical officers I had anything to do with. I just found him an honest, decent fellow who was out to do whatever he could to help people. Most of the doctors were good, John was outstanding.

When interviewed for this book Lloyd's cognitive faculties were sliding fast. His memories were patchy of his time as a doctor on the railway. That was, until he was shown a photograph—one in a book of George Aspinall's black and white photographs. When the first page fell open, nonagenarian Lloyd Cahill lunged forward, eyes sparkling: 'There it is! My old hospital!' He was referring to 'Cholera Hill, Shimo Sonkurai Camp number one'. It was hardly a hospital: just a couple of tents and a few bamboo structures. Lloyd pointed out the bamboo table where operations were performed, and the tent in which the dead bodies accumulated: 'We had to do all sorts of things; amputations, with no anaesthetic; they were just held down while we did it. The Japs—some of them were awful bastards. Cruel. They had no idea at all. We had nothing at all . . . we'd go out and find a dog and kill and cook the dog. I was down to about five and a half stone.' Then, just as quickly as he'd come to life, Lloyd sank back, his sudden recognition of his old camp on the railway surprising as it was moving to witness.

One of John's grim responsibilities, forced on him by the Japanese, was to vet suitable men for these labour camps; to cull from their ranks the men who were to be sent to work on the railway. It was a task he never forgot; it was, it seems—when we listen to his wife's recollections—a scar on his life for which he perhaps never entirely forgave himself. John was one of many doctors who fought for their men and tried to protect them from Japanese brutality. And, it is more than likely, he did so with his customary humility and courage. But years after the war, John was tormented by these men who'd left Changi under his authority, and returned wretched, if indeed they returned at all. Jean remembers her husband's anguish:

> My poor husband was horrified when he was asked to recom-
> mend people to work on building the railway. [At first] he
> thought he was sending them into the fresh air, but they were
> put in death camps and beaten and starved, and he felt he
> should have looked after those men better.

At various times John commanded the cookhouse. And when it came to nutrition he was a no-nonsense doctor.

> I was asked by the cooks to condemn a batch of rotten fish. I
> said 'You stupid bastards. We won't get any replacement.
> It's rich in protein and maggots. Thrash it within an inch of its
> long departed life, sieve out the bones and maggots and serve it
> as fish soup. It won't kill you but it will nourish you.'

There were numerous ways to try to replenish vitamins. The local grass—lalang—was a crude source of vitamin B. It was collected in armfuls with scythes and reaping hooks. Bundles of the grass were then churned in a mechanical device the engineers had scraped together from cannibalised metal found in the camp. From the outside the contraption looked a bit like a brickies' cement barrel. Inside, the grass clippings swirled about, shredded by a device that was a cross between a coffee grinder and a lawn mower. Out cranked a slurry of tens of thousands of gallons of liquid grass. The men detested its foul taste and often refused to drink it. John, smiling in remembrance, recalled that this grass soup 'was a light orange colour, rich in riboflavin and as bitter as hell. Known locally as "Tiger's piss", it helped, but not nearly enough.'

In spite of the huge effort that went into making 'Tiger's piss' and convincing the troops to drink it, hundreds of men were stalked by nutrition-related illnesses. As well as beri-beri and pellagra, men came down with painful rashes and skin fissures in just about every body crease imaginable. Some were plagued by the sensation of burning feet, and an illness called 'barbed-wire disease' that resulted in irritability, lassitude, depression and difficulty concentrating.

The doctors in Changi convinced their military chiefs that more should and could be done to prevent and treat nutritional deficiency diseases in the camp. What they came up with was well ahead of its time and, to this day, stands as an impressive example of captives using medical research to resist imprisonment and attempted extermination.

First, they calculated as precisely as possible the nutritional value of the foods available in Changi: including the very inadequate supplies provided by the Japanese and what little they passed on from the Red Cross; what the captives could scrounge through the black market; and what they produced themselves from grass and the like. Then they investigated the nutrient deficiency diseases and their occurrence in the camp to help them work out exactly what vitamins and minerals might be missing or out of balance in 'the rations'.

What they did then was almost unique for the times anywhere in the world, let alone in a prison camp. Throughout Changi, men were

divided into test and control groups and randomly assigned supplements like yeast in the form of Marmite, or vitamins in the form of
rice polishings, including the often-discarded outer coat of the grain.
The aim was to see what worked best. Walter Sarkies, an Australian
POW, captured the essence of these experiments in a cartoon. In
the process he implied that allocation of supplements may not have
been even-handed, with officers more likely than lower ranks to get
Marmite. Whatever the truth of the matter, discipline and organisation were critical in moulding and executing the plan and delivering
help to those in need.

One of the hospital wards, for the most seriously ill, went under
the facetious nickname, 'the fattening pen' and was reserved for
patients under six stone, John remembering that 'we used to try to
channel in little titbits to them'. At one point, when John was in
command of the cookhouse, it was his responsibility to escort the
sergeant of the cookhouse to make certain 'the goodies' didn't disap-
pear en route to 'the fattening pen'. On one such walk he observed,
unsentimentally, how the 'puppies of the Nip guards' were plopped
into this potpourri of food to enrich the miserable offerings. By then,
John was so inured to the hardship of life he thought nothing of this
delectable addition to his needy patients' food.

In later years, John often reflected on the bizarre items he
dropped into his mouth to survive as a POW: 'It's amazing what you
will eat when you are starving.' On one occasion he tried a banquet
of snails but gave them up: 'whatever you did to them they always
tasted like boot leather'. Outside the barbed perimeter of Changi,
the jungle teemed with wildlife, and although much was foreign
to Australian sensibilities, when wildlife was sliced and roasted,
few questions were asked. John took a fancy to snake. 'Some boys
brought back a small python after a scavenging expedition under
guard and gave me a 1 inch steak—delicious—just like chicken.'

Back at The Righi, as the war stretched on, Jean also made do with
whatever came to hand. It was not the only time life had been hard;

she'd known austerity before. Jean had grown up in Adelaide, the only daughter and youngest of four children, with chooks clucking and scratching about the backyard. She recollected stories from her childhood of how her grandmother chased down and decapitated chickens. When interviewed in 1999, Jean shuddered in remembrance:

> We kept them in the backyard for a few weeks; and we'd feed them up. My grandma, my mother's mother, could quite happily kill a chook and defeather it. Grandma evidently stretched its neck out along a board, and cut its head off.

With Christmas on the horizon, Jean knew that something special was expected; roast chicken for her boys would be ideal. So Jean set about the job of erecting a chook house in the backyard. She headed to the local hardware store and bought what she thought she needed: wire-netting, nails and planks of wood. She carted them by herself into the backyard and set about the unenviable task of construction. 'I had no one to build a little pen for the chooks; and I had no idea how anyone got a little fowl house to stand up, but I did have a paling fence . . . I did this with the aid of my Johnny looking over my shoulder.' Once her toil was done she bought a couple of chickens from Victoria market and waited.

As the days until Christmas diminished, her anxiety rose. Soon it would be time to slaughter a fowl. Vainly she tried to fortify her resolve with childhood memories, as if somehow her grandmother's act of slitting a chicken neck was a genetic gift passed on through the generations. Thinking she might yet get a reprieve she sought help from John's father but was dismissed with a surly: 'Make sure you do it properly. If you don't do it properly it will run around with its head off . . .' Jean, miserable, returned home and set about the act. 'I decided my boy Johnny shouldn't watch Mummy kill the chook, so I did it when he wasn't about.' Remembering how she grappled with the terrified frantic fowl, her voice breaks and mortified tears fall. 'I found it so very hard to hold . . . to get its silly head down . . .

but I did it. I did it. Do you know . . . I was crying out "Why should I have to do it!"'

The injustice of her lot tormented Jean during the war years, even in the tiniest of domestic tasks. 'Many a time I was wiping dishes, and one of the boys would ask for something. As simple as help turning on a tap. It was too hard, too stiff for their little hands. My eldest boy would be at the sink and call out, "I want a drink of water" and all I could think was "Somebody turn on the tap!"' Jean's silent screams went unheard during the war. Her war was waged in the kitchen and the backyard, imprisoned by circumstance and the perimeter of her Melbourne suburban home. At one point, seeking to atone for what she imagined as her gender deficit when it came to 'boy things', she tried her hand at building 'a little billycart . . . I'd got the tacks from the newsagent'. As she ruefully admitted, the tacks lay down rather than stayed upright. In winter she inexpertly 'tried to teach them how to kick a football. When John came home from the war he said: "but you don't kick like that" . . . apparently I kicked it with my toe . . . .' Her war was the loneliest of wars.

Jean's isolation and dread about her husband's fate was relieved only sparingly during John's five-year absence. She received just two postcards from him during his Changi incarceration: nothing more than the highly censored standardised lines that POWs were occasionally permitted to send. These mutilated cards made Jean's heart lurch. In some ways, receiving this desultory fare only sharpened her pain. 'I knew it was John's . . . the signature . . . no one could write John's signature. It was always so tidy. One just said, "I am well, John" . . . and the family went crazy. But I looked at the date and it was 15 months since it was sent. For all I knew my husband mightn't have been still alive.'

9

We know that John, sporadically, received letters from Jean during his Changi years, although, sadly, the whereabouts, or even the survival, of her letters is unknown. The evidence for John having received these letters comes in jottings he made in a small book he kept from this time. The book—*Easy Malay Vocabulary*—is pocket-sized and suitable for hiding and John's squiggles cram every corner, like graffiti on a billboard. It is a treasure-trove, telling us a lot about his Changi days.

The book itself is nothing much to look at. An unprepossessing volume, its canvas binding is frayed and its pastel blue cover stained with the damp and dirt of his years in Changi. The book remains a family favourite, preciously harboured by John's children, and today sits unobtrusively behind the glass pane of a book cabinet. A piece of paper is tucked inside. On it is written: 'Papa John's language book—full of card game scores with his fellow mates/prisoners. WW II, '41–'45.' And yes, he played card games; plenty of them, if the numbers of carefully lined pencil columns is anything to judge by. Bridge was his favourite game. But the book points to a lot more than casual pastimes.

This small book reveals John's mind as extraordinarily active. At one point he draws a detailed graph with about 30–40 vertical lines, crossed with another 30–40 horizontal lines—it is his form

of Changi graph paper. And then, as any secondary school mathematics student will see, he makes a series of calculations using a
geometric series. What was he nutting out? A problem of nutrition?
Then we find he has sketched a crude syringe—like a da Vinci sketch
of an unbuilt flying craft—with an internal coiled spring visible. It
looks all the world as if he might—using the cast-off bits and pieces
around him—construct such a syringe to use on his patients. John
was a handy man and could turn his hand to just about anything. A
syringe like this was a snap. Just as dire circumstance sharpened the
need for clinical observation in the absence of more formal investigations; so too did it sharpen the ingenuity of improvisation in
solving day-to-day problems of caring for sick men. John's syringe
was almost certainly just one of many ingenious ideas hard-pressed
men cranked out to survive.

At another point he draws what looks like a sophisticated water
tank, surrounded by lines of calculations. Perhaps a design for some
clandestine engineering project? Then, on another page, he details
the caloric value of porridge, bread, butter and jam. At first glance
it suggests the fantasies of a malnourished man, but more likely it is
evidence of John's involvement in the nutritional experiments undertaken in Changi. His writing remains crisp and precise. Despite his
malnutrition and at times vitamin-bleached brain, his measured
hand remains the same.

On page 122, we come across an unexpected passage. He writes:

Overjoyed getting your December message. Keeping well,
working Hedley's [Col. Hedley Summons, an Australian officer
and a close friend of John's who was appointed head of Roberts
Hospital during 1942] hospital with old friends. Fondest love to
you sweetheart. Daddy's dear boys, parents, brothers, friends.

So it looks like he'd just received a letter from Jean. And when he
read it, he thanked his God and tucked it 'lovingly in [his] breast
pocket'.

The knowledge that the Japanese were losing the war was invaluable to the POWs; this life-sustaining information came to them via radio. They just needed the odd wireless here and there to pick up the news. John, towards the end of his life, recalled the importance of knowing what was happening in the war outside Changi:

> After the Battle of the Coral Sea in about April 1942 we knew that Australia was safe and after the Battle of Midway . . . we knew that Japan was doomed . . . The reason for this was that we had secret radios operating throughout and marvels of ingenuity they were. One was hidden in the head of a wooden broom. On another occasion a young soldier came up to me and asked whether I could lay my hands on a spare stethoscope.

The stethoscope was to listen to the soft broadcast of a wireless interred in the cavity of a wall, away from prying Japanese eyes and ears. What John—circumspect and unassuming—did not mention was his own exceptional bravery in dispersing the news received by the concealed radios. For the full story on how John did this, we have Private Bill Flowers to thank.

In surviving Changi photographs, Bill Flowers stands in the sun like a sapling, an overly tall soldier, bare-chested and all toothy smiles under a slouch hat. He looks like the kid next door, because that's exactly what he was. He spent most of his time working in and around the hospital, so he knew John Cade intimately. John's bravery in dispensing the BBC radio news left an indelible trace on Bill's mind. This is how Bill tells it:

> John was eventually second in command of the unit . . . a great officer. He wasn't a demanding type of person but had the ability to get things done . . . now we weren't permitted to have radios. But there were secret radios in Changi that were operated from which BBC news then could be spread around the camp. John would bring us this news.
>
> John Cade used to travel from the hospital area in Changi, which was at Roberts Barracks to headquarters . . . which

meant going through one access gate in the wire at the hospital, travelling along the road to the headquarters area, past Japanese guard posts. One would never know when one might be stopped . . . and might be searched. John Cade used to come back with notes on the BBC news . . .

We would gather on the top floor of a two storey building and he would recount it . . . I can remember it so clearly . . . John delivered the news just as though he was the BBC news announcer himself . . . he did it, maybe, several times a week . . . you had to be careful how all this was done. We'd have our lookouts—'cockatoos'—posted and John used to read out the news but then came a time when it was too dangerous to bring it back on paper . . . and so he committed it to memory.

If you were searched and found to have notes on you . . . if you were found out. Well, obviously the Kempei Tai . . . that's the Jap military police . . . you'd be put in prison . . . there were fellows who had fallen foul of the Japanese, and they then received terrible treatment . . . It was very dangerous carrying the BBC news . . .

————

John's view about the cause of mental symptoms was profoundly influenced by his time in Changi. He kept a record of his 'mental ward' cases, and, what is more, he wrote at least one report summarising his observations. So in the midst of war and malnutrition and the hideous deformity of what is good in humanity, the wheels of organisation continued to whir: 'I had ample time to meditate on the possible causes [of serious mental illnesses such as manic depression] and plan some sort of research programme for when the fruitful years might return. I certainly did not come up with any specific hypotheses but these could be regarded as germinal years.' And there is no doubt that John's thinking about the cause of illnesses such as manic depression underwent a radical change. Fortunately for us, he described a series of cases in which the evolution of his thinking can be reconstructed to some degree.

Two of these cases left a deep impression on John. The first was of an intrepid young soldier with 'a very gallant battle record'. Soon after captivity in Changi, this young soldier's mind unravelled. He dissolved into an untameable manic state of excitability, restless activity and utter irresponsibility. As John looked into the eyes of this young soldier, he made the diagnosis of a manic phase of manic depression. He looked, for all the world, like one of the patients incarcerated in Beechworth. And then, unexpectedly, this young soldier dropped dead. John immediately performed an autopsy. What he found astounded him. The soldier had 'the biggest chronic subdural haematoma' John had ever seen, 'the size of a partly deflated football'.

A subdural haematoma is an abnormal collection of blood wedged between the brain and the skull. It is a kind of bruising of the brain, caused by trauma to the head. As the blood collects it exerts pressure on the brain and alters human behaviour. In this case, it caused the soldier's manic state. Somewhere in the recent past this soldier, probably in the last days of battle, had suffered a head injury. It was enough to start the bleeding between the brain and skull, but it took some time for the symptoms to develop. And when they did, he became manic. Years later, John wrote carefully of this story as one of his salutary lessons in medical life, teaching him the pitfalls of drawing conclusions before obtaining all the available evidence.

The second case was of a medical orderly room sergeant who complained that his hearing was failing. Next his body became 'spastic', which in neurological circles means his muscle tone increased to the point where he might lose control of bodily movements. This increase in muscle tone might result in bizarre uncoordinated muscle contractions such as coarse tremors and a stiff gait. At first glance, such a man might be suspected of fabricating an illness. In this light, John, who was called in to consult on the sergeant, at first wondered if this might be a picture of hysteria. Hysteria was the diagnosis psychiatrists made when a patient presented to them with an apparent physical illness—such as paralysis of the legs or a bizarre gait—but where the cause was purely psychological. Like the first patient, the sergeant died suddenly. At his autopsy, his central nervous system revealed a loss of myelin—the protective coating around the nerves—a condition that also occurs in multiple sclerosis. John knew immediately that the cause of this sergeant's odd presentation had nothing to do with psychiatry; it had all to do with an abnormality in his spinal nerves.

These two cases—the 'manic' soldier and the uncoordinated 'hysterical' sergeant—stuck in John's mind for the rest of his medical career. The notion that mental symptoms were somehow anchored to an underlying physical or chemical problem was one John kept coming back to. He later wrote that 'I could see that so many of the psychiatric patients suffering from [illnesses such as manic depression and schizophrenia] appeared to be sick people in the medical sense. This fired my ambition to discover their aetiology.'

This single distilled idea—that mental illness should be seen in the same light as physical illness—foreshadowed much of John Cade's future work. It was an idea that kindled gently in his mind. And, once accepted by him, the verity of this finding never faded.

———

On 6 August 1945 the Americans dropped an atomic bomb on Hiroshima, then another on 9 August, obliterating Nagasaki; six days after Nagasaki the Japanese unconditionally surrendered.

In the days after surrender, John's throat tightened with the fear that he, along with his fellow POWs, might be executed before they were rescued. And, just for a moment, his immaculate composure wobbled. In one of his letters home he wrote of this uncertain period: 'One of our worst fears . . . [was] . . . that [the Japanese] would never let us be recaptured alive if it came to a fight to the finish.' Three decades later he recalled these 'final frightening few days' when he and several other POWs 'planned a last funk hole—up a sewer with three days' supplies'. As it turned out John's survival plans were thankfully not needed and, surprisingly, the Japanese acquiesced with little bloodshed. After three and a half years, John Cade was about to walk free.

Newly liberated, John furiously set about writing letters to Jean. He carefully marked the number 100 at the top of the first page of the first letter; and reminded himself that his last letter, number 99, was penned before capitulation in February 1942. He wrote letter after letter, pouring everything into this cathartic act. Some were posted singly; others despatched in batches. And he waited, anxiously, for Jean's first letter to arrive.

Re-reading these letters, we feel his urgency to make up for stolen time—what the children might look like, what presents they might like—and we understand his need to please and surprise them. But his deepest doubt was that he may somehow fail them. That, somehow, five years of war may have filleted out the best of what he was, leaving just the leftovers. Several times his anxieties surfaced when writing about his two boys, Jack and David: 'How I look forward to smiling into those two eager young faces, and how I hope that the real daddy does not fall short by too far, of their dream daddy.' In these darker moments, self-doubt, the assassin of dreams, took root in John's mind.

He was also very anxious to make sure Jean was aware that he had survived:

> we still have no assurance that you have been notified that we
> are alive and well . . . . It has been a horrible anxiety for you, far
> more than for me because I have been reasonably sure that you
> have been all right whereas you knew almost nothing about me.

He repeatedly reassures Jean about his physical state, as if dispelling her concerns that somehow he might have been damaged or is no longer the man she married—the deep and disturbing dread of all returning married POWs.

In other moments, John swells with the anticipation of coming home, and lets fantasy run wild. 'Making up for this lost time. I've thought and dreamed and planned about that glorious holiday that

you and I and the kiddies are going to have . . .' He dreams of going
to a restaurant with Jean and slicing into a prime cut of beef, 'a
porterhouse steak at Flosie's'.

In his final weeks in Changi, John kneels at the altar to receive
the sacrament and gives thanks for his salvation: 'It has been possible
to go to Holy Communion for the first time since Easter (owing to
the shortage of altar bread) and I have been daily from Sunday until
today (Thursday) . . . kneeling in adoration and thankfulness to Our
Lord.' Several times in these early letters home he stops short of
more brutal descriptions of his captors, implying that these words
can wait. But every now and then a moment of fury overwhelms him
and it penetrates his conversation:

> our long deferred Red Cross Supplies are being brought in and
> distributed—supplies that had been held up indefinitely by the
> incredibly grasping, corrupt Japanese administration. The Jap
> war machine is the foulest most soulless thing ever invented by
> the wickedness of man . . . it blisters my soul when I dwell on
> it . . .

Over the previous five years there had been small hard-won
victories of life over death. From now on, nothing was to be
wasted; particularly time. Reflectively, he wrote: 'I believe all of us
consciously or unconsciously have a much better sense of values,
and a greatly enhanced appreciation of the good things in life.' John
developed a deep affection for the local Chinese population, doing
'a wonderful job in Malaya throughout the Japanese occupation,
spying, sabotaging, non-cooperating'. At war's end it was decided
that the AIF would come up with something, perhaps an award, to
honour the local Chinese population for their bravery and sacri-
fice. John proposed that a scholarship fund be set up to support
local nurses in Malaya to travel to Australia, and was, later, deeply
involved in administering it. Called the AIF Malayan Nursing
Scholarship, it is the official war memorial of the AIF who served
in Malaya.

Almost a month after the Japanese surrender, John was yet to leave the camp, still working as a doctor as the number of sick and injured swelled to record levels.

And then he writes, '[I] hope to go in tomorrow to take three British officers (mental cases) to the British hospital ship'. The following day John took his first steps outside the camp. He escorted the psychiatrically disturbed British officers to their ship—one senior RAF officer with a manic condition travelled home in 'a steel-mesh cage'. Singapore, John reflected as he walked through the remnants of a city obliterated by an orgy of violence, was a city 'of the dead. The Nips have apparently not had any repairs done to buildings—you see decay and inattention everywhere, gardens overrun with weeds ... crumbling walls, shuttered shops.' Soon after, John took his first dip in the sea and was repeatedly stung by a jellyfish; but he was a hardened man by then and nothing could detract from the moment of joy. Especially, he writes, 'with not a Nip on the horizon to mar the scene'.

There was one moment in these giddy days of emancipation that marked John's transition from captive to free man. It occurred while he walked through the smoking ruins of Singapore. Looking to the skies, his eyes caught a shimmer of iridescent blue ascending above the city. A kingfisher, the shade of sapphire, streaked by—John's 'first glimpse of beauty' in over three years.

Even then John was mindful not to allow his spirits to swing wildly. Changi had changed John; he had learned well the survival skill of never allowing emotions to spill over, of not allowing his facial expression to betray his thoughts. Uncontrolled emotions could be misunderstood, and John was always mindful of the presence of Japanese guards who might respond with violence. Controlling one's emotions was a skill needed to stay alive. His deep-seated reserve would confuse some people in the post-war years when trying to assess John Cade.

Changi changed John in many ways, but one thing Changi could not break was John's addiction to tobacco. Rapturously, on liberation, he wrote home to Jean of his first pack of Camel cigarettes, 'I inhaled it all the way down to my G-string.'

At war's end Jean dashed off a telegram and a letter to friends—Dr Frank Prendergast and his wife, Lil, living at Claremont Mental Hospital, Perth—capturing the moment of joy. The scribbled and obviously hastily sent telegram, stamped 12 September 1945, stated in staccato words: 'John's name radio today Singapore list write when official.' Jean had finally heard on the radio that John had survived.

And she does write to them, one week later:

Gosh! I hardly know how to start . . . my hand and mind is rather unsteady . . . *Yesterday* two letters one dated 6th and one 10th Sept. By his handwriting and the way he expressed himself I could tell he was well and had not changed one bit . . . His writing is tidy and well controlled as of old—he is as loving as ever . . . The phone here and at Bundoora has hardly stopped ringing since last Wednesday . . . We have been told that Beechworth, Sunbury, Mont Park and Bundoora are agog . . . The children are so sweet, they gave me tremendous hugs as Daddy's letter told them to do. The other morning about 5 am David heard a plane and wondered if Daddy would be in it. He seemed to think John might parachute down. Our house has been painted and garden tidied.

As John steamed back from Singapore on the cargo vessel *Largs Bay* in the September of 1945, he took pen to paper and wrote these prescient lines to his wife:

Then to work—as you guessed in one of your early letters the old brain box is simmering with ideas. I believe this long period of waiting has allowed many of my notions in psychiatry to crystallise, and I'm just bursting to put them to the test. If they work out, they would represent a great advance in the knowledge of 'manic-depressive' insanity and primary dementia [schizophrenia]—sounds like my usual over-optimism, doesn't it?! Well, there is only one way to find out—test it and see.

And then, on Friday 28 September, 'Tomorrow will be a great day for us—Australia!'

————————

John's two boys have their own distinct memories of waiting for their father. Jack was turning seven and David just five. Their memories, although rusty in patches, still cling to them; Jack's recollections are more restrained than his younger brother's:

> Mum didn't know if Dad was alive or dead towards the end of the war. She had very limited information. I recall her telling us that he was on his way home . . . she was probably scared as to what he was like if he was still viable, the man she knew . . . she didn't want to raise expectations.

David's memory, no doubt mingled with what he has absorbed from family stories over the years, evokes the moment of anxiety and anticipation, common in so many Australian households huddled round radios at war's end:

> I remember the radio quite clearly . . . it was about a foot high and a foot and a half wide and was timber framed, with a dial which the vertical pointer moved along. It had a circular vent at the top with a couple of grill bars, cloth mesh . . . I don't remember what we listened to during the war but I do remember that we were sitting on the floor in the small lounge room listening to the radio when peace was declared . . .
>
> Mum was listening to the names of POWs on the *Largs Bay* vessel . . . And they were reading out the names in alphabetical order and we heard Dad's name read out . . .

David can reach back into time and recall further snippets from those heady post-war days—how his mother always had her hair in a bun the size of a squashed tennis ball and wore floral dresses, always neat and clean, even if she did not own many. Somehow these visible attributes fixed themselves in David's young mind, and, closing his eyes, he describes the scene as if lived today. Jean, he went on, was quiet at the time of the announcement, not demonstrative; relief in her husband's homecoming was something she savoured silently and, we have no doubt, with bountiful prayer.

———

During the Changi years, the thought of meeting his wife and two boys was John's most cherished desire; it was also his most feared. Jean was cut from a stoic cloth—he could count on her, no matter how affected and worn by war he appeared. But his children? That was another matter. He barely knew them; Jack was little more than a toddler and David was a baby in Jean's arms when he walked away from their home in January 1941. It was now almost five years later. They would be strangers to him, but even more so, he knew he would be a stranger to them.

On his return to Melbourne John was met by his parents, who whisked him off immediately to the Repatriation Hospital in Heidelberg, where he was treated for malnourishment and bronchitis. Jean and the two boys were to meet him there.

As Jean and the two boys stood in the hospital hallway, a gaunt, yellow-faced, dressing-gowned apparition approached. Jean and the boys can still remember the exchange of words as John tentatively came towards his children.

'I seem to recall mum saying, "This is your dad",' remembers Jack. 'Is that really my dad, I wondered?' If he had doubts, he was old enough and diplomatic enough to keep his lips clipped. That couldn't be said for his younger brother David, always the more voluble of the two.

David, wide-eyed and disbelieving, bellowed, 'Mummy, that's not my daddy! How do I know he's my daddy?'

Jack, older and wiser, countered, 'I know he's my daddy because I can remember him coming to our place with a little wooden train set.'

David replied, 'But his teeth are all black!'

When the scenario of exchanges is replayed for David today, he laughs. The images he had of his father were formed by those he saw around the house—of a well-nourished, fit young man in uniform: 'When I saw him my mental picture was of the photos I'd seen before the war . . . I thought that this chap walking down the corridor towards us didn't look at all like him, and I hid behind Mum.'

Jean was true to form—calm and undemonstrative, measured and loving. She managed John and the boys because no one else could. Privately she was dismayed by her husband's appalling appearance, made worse by skin made yellow by the anti-malarial drug Atebrin: 'I could hardly recognise him myself. He looked dreadful; his knee bones stuck out from the opening in his dressing gown. I remember when he came home, his nose was just bone, and his skin was horrible . . . it was the first thing I saw, his hollowed face . . . he looked as though he'd been starved.'

Although she was desperate for John to share his experiences of the previous five years, he was steadfast in resisting. 'He said he didn't want to talk about his experiences, he just wanted to come home.' All she extracted from John, at least initially, was that it was 'a terrible time . . . anything you'd want to know . . . the men wouldn't talk about it . . . but he was the same lovely personality . . . gentle . . . there was no anger'.

In the decades afterwards, John referred to his time in Changi as the 'interminable' years, that seemingly eternal time of suffering. John was about to turn 34. He was angry that war had stolen from him the finest years of his professional life, and fearful that it had robbed him of his finest years with his two young children.

Although weakened, John resolved to resume his psychiatric work as quickly as possible. As Jean recollected:

he was . . . longing to get back to work . . . he was wanting to get going, to get started . . . When he came home from Changi one of the first things he said to me: 'I must get busy, I've spent five years away; three and a half years as a prisoner of war and I had to look after people with no equipment . . . I must find something to stop the melancholy.'

John knew the awful sight of the melancholic patient, severely depressed, sitting mute and immobile, tormented by black thoughts of death; he also knew of other patients who roared and spun into a kind of celestial mania. It was to these extremes of mood that John turned his mind as he prepared to return to asylum life.

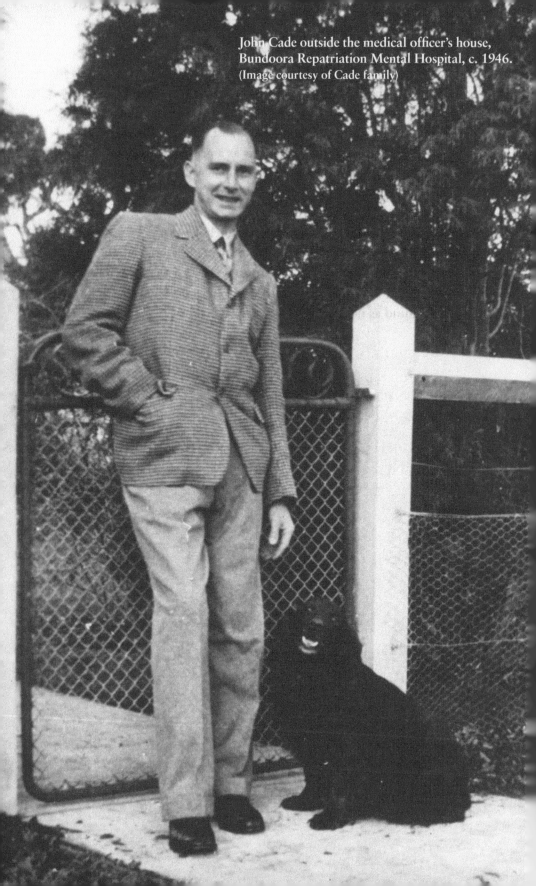

PART 3

Salt *of* *the* Earth

A TREATMENT FOR MANIA:
The prolonged bath

[The bath] is given at a temperature of about 98° to 100° F. It has a marked effect on maniacal patients. It is given daily, and . . . prolonged from day to day until a patient may remain in the bath for four or five hours . . . Some authorities use a lid to the bath with a hole in it, through which the head of the patient projects.

Handbook for Mental Nurses, *7th edition, 1941*

JOHN CADE: *On experimentation*

For goodness sake don't waste your time elaborating untestable hypotheses. Guessing becomes merely a game unless it is a plan for action.

...he question of scrap iron for Japan, right enough...

...was going to be done with it.

...that this Indonesian bid for independence is only...
...read dissatisfaction by the peoples of the East wi...
...ver lordship. The same problem is demanding solu...
...Burma and Indo-China...

...n of political speculation. Regarding leave, des...
...ut at 28 days immediately following disembar...
...k or so in a convalescent camp (probably at Bal...
...l over-haul, followed by another 30 days leave...
...are not sure of yet is whether we will get i...
...cumulated recreation leave which would amo...
...70-80 days. I suppose the department will...
...me as soon as possible, - well, they will have...
...and I, darling, are entitled to a pretty good...
...that, I feel so rusty medically, that I simp...
...if possible three months post-graduate stud...
...like to do a month at St Vincents, a month at...
...a fortnight at the Eye and Ear, leaving a mo...
...swinging. - all provided we can keep the depar...
...her to work - as you guessed in one of your l...
...old brain box is simmering with ideas. I be...
...riod of waiting has allowed many of my no...
...try to crystallise, and I'm just bursting to p...
...test. If they work out, they would represent a...
...the knowledge of...

10

Bundoora Repatriation Mental Hospital, nearly twenty kilometres to the north of Melbourne, was set on a rise on the landscape, visible to all, yet cut off from the currents of normal life. It was a hospital in character and rhythm, more rural than urban, and by the late 1940s it spread over 160 acres, with over 50 scattered buildings and just on 200 ex-diggers filling its wards and roaming its expansive grounds.

This elevated plot of land was at once the highest point in metropolitan Melbourne and a world in itself, amputated from normal society. But it had not always been so. And the clue to its oncesplendid past lay at the very heart of the asylum.

At that heart stood Ward A, which housed the more manageable convalescing men: men who, while not ready to rip the place apart, were still troubled by fantasies of the mind. Some slept on the ground floor; others made their way up the broad sweeping staircase and slept on the first floor, out on the spacious verandah with a view of the Melbourne skyline.

In the 1940s, even with a cursory look, one would have sensed that this imposing building—defaced by tacky renovations—had once been a magnificent homestead. But when John returned to Bundoora in 1946, Ward A was a shabby, blemished parody of itself: its wide first-floor verandah enclosed by canvas; cheap timbers nailed on the outside; ornaments cracked, broken or stolen; the divine, oval stained-glass skylight, under which nurses could recall dancing with ex-servicemen, blackened with grime and panels cracked.

Forty years earlier, Ward A had been the famed 'Bundoora Homestead', an architectural masterpiece in Queen Anne revivalist style, designed and constructed in 1899 for the very wealthy Mr John Matthew Vincent Smith, known in horse-racing circles simply as J.V.

Smith made his mansion and its surrounds into one of the finest horse studs in the Commonwealth. An equine empire, the Bundoora stud was a name famous throughout the nation. It was here that the virile stallion Wallace, the first son of Carbine, grazed and sired. Of course, all Australians knew of Carbine, the legendary winner of the 1890 Melbourne Cup in record time, and with the heaviest weight ever recorded: a superstar not rivalled in human form. The chestnut Wallace was not far behind. His wins included the Caulfield Guineas, Victoria Derby and Sydney Cup. But he is best remembered as a sire. His progeny galloped the grounds of Bundoora and went on to win two Melbourne Cups and six Victoria Derbys. In its pomp, Bundoora was a horse-lover's paradise and a place to be seen for the fashionable folk of Edwardian Melbourne.

In 1920, Smith sold his home and the estate to the Commonwealth Government and the fate of the homestead turned. It would be converted into a convalescent farm to accommodate and restore those soldiers who returned, mentally damaged, from the First World War. The Bundoora estate, once a masculine empire of the finest bloodlines, would now, ironically, accept discarded men, seeking to reinvigorate them.

In the years after the First World War, thousands of men returned to Melbourne with minds broken, unable to resume their previous lives. Bundoora would change all that, or so it was hoped. The *Argus* newspaper reported that these 'war derelicts' could be regenerated. In gushing tones, suggestive of an advertisement for a modern-day health retreat, *The Argus* enthused that Bundoora was 'charmingly situated a few miles beyond Preston, and adjacent to the Macleod sanatorium for TB soldiers . . . The sight of these wrecked soldiers, patiently graduating from simple jobs, such as tending flower gardens, to the more arduous duties of the farm labourer, is gratifying and inspiring.'

One might just imagine an old-fashioned Movietone newsreel in black and white, flickering with romantic images of beaming returned diggers pruning azalea bushes for the cameras, and the sound blaring gratuitous homilies in a nasal Aussie twang: 'And here we have our returned heroes; once damaged, now clipping their way back into society.' Some even managed to do so.

Some men at the Mental Hospital recuperated for relatively short stints, others for life. Visitors came—sometimes bringing afternoon teas—to see husbands, brothers and fathers; but they did not visit in the profusion one might expect. Visiting hours in the late 1940s were limited and reflected the regimentation of hospital life. And, regardless of these bureaucratic matters, the mentally ill were regarded, at large, with ambivalence. Some families—embarrassed or just wanting to forget—simply faded from view. It was to this place— once a haven for the wealthy in their bright silk frockcoats and now a refuge for forgotten men—that John returned, living quietly with his family without too much to disturb them.

John, Jean and the boys moved into the squat single-storey red-brick bungalow reserved for the resident doctor. The front of the house looked away from the hospital wards in roughly a westerly direction, towards sprawling paddocks that trailed downwards several kilometres to a narrow gully with a creek.

The back of the house faced the hospital wards, and it was through a gate in the back fence and along a gently coiling gravel path that John walked each day to see his patients. He returned in the late afternoon by the same gate, rarely bothering to enter the house via the front door. The doctor's house was as much a part of the asylum as any of the wards in which the patients lived.

Perhaps the most famous photograph we have of John Cade, and certainly the most endearing, is from these early post-war years at Bundoora. In the photo he stands next to the wrought-iron front gate of his house. We get no glimpse of the house in the photo but the surrounds—a thicket of trees and a timber post supporting a chicken wire fence—suggest a rustic setting. As for John himself, his methodical mien is reflected in the sharply folded creases that run midline down each of his trouser legs, his tightly buttoned tweed jacket that compresses and conceals his war-time-wasted chest, and his hair, gently receding, greased to the point of glistening and combed back hard. A naturally lean man, he bends slightly, awkwardly, to one side and has a hand in his coat pocket. He seems a trifle embarrassed. Nonetheless, he does his best with a self-conscious smile. The more relaxed figure in the photograph is Peter, the cocker spaniel, who presents a classic pose and eyes the camera without flinching.

The timeless photograph of John taken outside his Bundoora house betrays his attention to hairstyle—not a wayward strand of hair is visible. To maintain this standard, he left the grounds of the asylum every 3–4 weeks for his favourite barber—Milburn's, in the suburb of Ivanhoe. And for shaving, long gone was his wartime moustache, but he'd kept a small ablutionary memento from his three and a half years of Japanese incarceration in Changi: his enamel shaving mug. In this mug he lathered to full bloom his camel hair brush for the finest of shaves.

As for his sons' hair, now that was another matter altogether. Haircuts for the boys were considered an extravagance in these years of austerity after the war. John Cade therefore decided that he would learn the art of cutting hair. So he sat and watched as the boys went for their regular haircuts, and diligently observed in that Cade way—deeply, finely, taking note of every implement and their application. With insatiable curiosity, he deluged the barber with questions. David recalled the event: 'He took us to the barber and, I remember, he learned how to do it from the barber. Afterwards he went and bought a pair of clippers.' The barber, apparently, was more than happy to assist, perhaps delighted that his adroitness with comb and scissor had an admirer. From that moment on John cut the boys' hair.

Expensive tastes—not only hair grooming—were clipped wherever and whenever possible in the Bundoora years, and in no area was this clearer than in his care for his sons' shoes. John kept a 'last', something that we might regard as anachronistic in the modern household garage, but a common appliance in the 1940s. A last is a solid model of a human foot around which a shoe is placed in readiness to be repaired. With this, he resoled and repaired the boys' shoes. His toolkit, lovingly kept from boyhood, contained everything he needed, including a shoemaker's hammer. It was just the type of detailed mechanical task he loved to perform. The boys remember their father, the psychiatrist, bent over a pair of school shoes gently and systematically tapping each tack into place.

––––––––

John Cade lived as he'd always done: routines were strictly followed. Not that he was a martinet; far from it. But there was a disciplined manner in which he conducted his life. Something he'd undoubtedly had before the war, but infinitely sharpened by it. Before each meal John said grace, and 'went to mass every Sunday if it was at all possible if he wasn't sick or the car hadn't broken down'. And at bedtime he'd kneel beside the boys and say prayers with them. And his good night statement was one that did not change: 'Good night, dear. Jesus, Mary and Joseph watch over you.'

Two further rituals, already embedded in his life, marked him out.

Cigarettes were smoked with reverence; they were the timepiece by which he carved up his day. At Bundoora, he smoked exactly seven cigarettes daily, but they were strategic: one at breakfast, morning tea, lunch, afternoon tea, dinner and two in the evening. Bought from his local barber, his favourites were cork-tipped Ardath cigarettes; he regarded the more common Turf cigarettes as just that.

Another ritual by which he set his day's chronometer was tea drinking. John drank Robur tea, 'routinely having two cups of scalding tea with sugar after breakfast'. And in parallel with his cigarettes, he had another two cups for morning tea, two for lunch, two with afternoon tea and another two at night after his evening meal. Each day he returned from the wards with military precision for morning and afternoon tea, and lunch.

John did a final round of his patients each evening. He'd leave via the back door, pass through his backyard and out the gate that stepped directly on to the asylum grounds, stopping along the way to take in the different pines and eucalypts on the grounds and the birds that rested in them, and keeping a sharp watch for the brown and tiger snakes that lurked in the tussocks on warm evenings. His inquisitive eye saw the world about him as sharply as he did his patients: what made a shrub flourish in certain locations, which ones prospered, and which ones faltered. He delighted in tracking the droppings of wildlife and was a self-confessed scatological special-ist. He was known by everyone—his wife, his children, patients, nurses and other staff—to halt at various points as he wandered the grounds and bend over something that had arrested his attention, and study it with an absorbed fixation, returning home with a wry observation about his find. It would not be long before patients came to the house to take a closer look at their nature-loving doctor.

II

When a shiny new doctor arrived at the hospital, the patients were always curious. So it was not long before an elderly digger nosed through the back fence gate—a porous filter at best—and offered to assist Jean: '"Hello missus, you got a lot of dishes there, would you like me to come and wash the dishes?" And so I let him come and wash my dishes.'

Next a weather-beaten old man came visiting. He moved about the paddocks in perpetual motion, gathering cow manure in bags to sprinkle on the Cade garden. One day, when the rain thumped down with biblical might upon the earth, the Cades saw him fossicking about, filling his bag. When he knocked at the front door, dripping and sodden and clutching his cow dung bag, he offered his smelly fertiliser but resisted all enticement to come in and dry himself.

Other patients filed past the house with sacks in their hands, like motley work gangs. They came to the front door offering mushrooms from their filthy sacks: 'Look what I've got for you, missus.' They went out of their way to offer their modest harvest. Why they did this may have been out of generosity, or gratitude, or, perhaps, because life offered so little social interaction that they took what they could.

As well as dish-washers, and cow dung and mushroom collectors, there was a haphazard trickle of curious and well-meaning men—old and young—in and out of the Cade bungalow, offering their services and food and whatever they thought the young doctor and his family might like.

––––––––––

The Bundoora asylum was a world within a world and, like all mental hospitals of the period, an infectious lassitude stretched out across its wards and grounds—a plodding attachment to doing things as they had been done in asylums for over a century.

Inside the wards, where the patients slept at night, beds were crammed against one another, thin rectangles wedged compactly. At night, some patients were compelled to clamber over one another if they needed assistance. It was a feat of endurance for so many psychotic and melancholic and war-damaged men to abide one another's company in such a fashion.

If you took the time to watch these men, you might observe that one thing unified them. They lived life in their own worlds and shuffled about like pilgrims awaiting a destination. From afar the asylum gave the illusion of a social community. But, in reality, each man was alone. Withdrawing into themselves and imprisoned by illness—whose disfigurement was unseen—they barely communicated with one another. Each man, in his own way, was a wreck. This was not a community of men; it was 200 communities.

Some men scowled at the torments that tugged at their minds; others waved their hands about, arguing with tree stumps. A few saw the outside world as a threat and stood alone, with eyes half-averted, whenever a stranger entered the grounds. The occasional catatonic man assumed an erect, rigid stance, a remnant of a military past. Some stalked about with arms akimbo, faces worn and surly; others sat on their haunches in a row, perched on a step.

Patients dressed themselves in a manner that hinted at a life beyond the asylum, and the longer the admission, the more dilapidated the clothing. For the most part, nothing fitted; and, colour, so absent in their lives, was also missing from their apparel. Their clothing was a nod to the times—formal and heavy—and mirrored a suffocating post-war Melbourne. The men wore street clothes of the day: often this was a jacket made of tweed, usually a waistcoat, a dress shirt and no tie. Boots were mandatory, socks were optional: the spit and polish of military boots were long gone. Leather belts, stripped of their buckles, were wrapped around the men's waists and tied into a knot to hold up sagging trousers. Those without belts found twine and used this instead. Patients wore grey felt hats any time of the day or year. In summer, corks dangled from strings attached to the brim to keep the flies away. For those patients unable to find a hat, grimy handkerchiefs with small knots tied in each corner mantled their heads.

The Cades embraced the patients, with all their oddities, as an extended family rather than as strangers. That warm relationship is our great stroke of good fortune. For the best and most intimate portrayal of these patients can only be found by living with them. And of all the Cades it was the two boys—Jack and David—who played and mingled with these men and who saw them with uncensored eyes. It is through the boys' memories that we have a rare window into asylum life. 'Certainly we knew they were loopy. But that was perfectly within the acceptable range for us.'

'Our friends called Bundoora the loony bin. But to us it was home, the patients our friends.'

Their schoolmates came over on weekends, riding around the hospital grounds on bikes; Jack and David got around on horseback: 'Jack rode a pony called Betty,' explains David. 'McCurdy got us the horses; he was just a grateful patient. McCurdy was allowed out, went to the pound and brought us back these horses. My horse was Kate, a fat draught horse. She was so broad I couldn't fit on a normal saddle. I'd plonk about with my legs splayed on the top.

'We learned a lot about the patients, these lovely people whose brains had gone. Lovely old guys, some a bit strange, some a lot strange, most completely lost. The hospital was their home; it was also ours.'

The boys knew the patients well, in that kind of way young boys who live in a world of their own making—partly supervised by parents but largely on the loose—are wont to do. It was a world often real, sometimes make-believe. The vague but undeniable anxiety adults felt when walking on the asylum grounds was never felt by the boys, and in some ways, the world the two Cade boys inhabited gave them an understanding of patients no adult could ever have. 'We weren't ever scared of them; only of the snakes, which slithered in the paddocks.'

To the north of the hospital one could see Mount Macedon and to the southwest, the grey skyline of Melbourne, flat and sluggish. But it was to the other points of the compass that the boys found most joy.

The paddocks extended to the west of the house a good distance down to the blackberry-lined creek. To the southeast the boys could walk or ride their horses across Plenty Road and into another asylum—Mont Park Mental Hospital. They spent plenty of time at Mont Park, where they played on the narrow train line that brought in coal to power the asylum's lights and heat its water and ovens, and larked about the Aboriginal canoe tree not far from the superintendent's house. The farm at Mont Park provided fresh fruit and vegies to Bundoora, and was a target for the boys: 'Jack and I would raid the orchard. You'd get pears, peaches, apricots and more.' Each day, a select group of Bundoora patients headed to Mont Park to work in the orchard, then helped transport food and milk back to Bundoora. 'The patients milked the cows at Mont Park and then they delivered the milk on horse and cart, originally in big billies that were about a metre high.'

Wide-eyed, the two boys came across individual patients that they remember to this day. Although the minds of the men they encountered overflowed with odd ideas and strangeness, there was a spot, here and there, like an oasis, where their past lives sat unscathed. Some of them were lettered men with the finest of educations; others were blessed with exquisite craft skills. One such man was Harry, a wizard with his hands. The boys took a shine to him. David recalls that, 'Harry was a genius at making things; he had a shed.' And it was into this wondrous shed that the boys disappeared, to be shown the magic of dismantling and mantling everything. Harry was their teacher and he could fix anything the boys brought to him.

Jack also remembers the patient well:

> Harry was an expert fixer of clocks and watches. You'd walk up a couple of timber steps and into, well, it was like an old-fashioned shop, his shed; it had lots of cogwheels. He taught me how to build a crystal set radio. I used to get spare parts from army disposals. I could easily still put together the small radio he taught me to make; I tucked it into an old cigarette box. I could pick up a few of the Melbourne radio stations: 3LO, 3AR, 3DB and I'd listen to the footy on Saturdays.

Frankie was another favourite of the boys. He'd sit outside the Cade house, in his three-piece suit minus a tie, and move about, cutting a bit of grass here and there. Frankie was a master of the obscure line and repeated endlessly—to no one in particular—one sentence: 'I'm just going to try and secure my observances.' Naturally no one had the remotest idea what Frankie was on about, but this lack of understanding seemed not to perturb him or them. Jack recalled some vital instructions Frankie imparted to the boys: 'He had a little chat with us, to show us how to smoke a cigarette. David and I used to collect butts from around the asylum and then you'd break them open and put them into the bowl of a clay pipe. Appalling stuff.'

In that respect the asylum was no different to the outside world: nearly everyone smoked. Tobacco, it seemed, was more coveted than discharge from the hospital. Cigarettes, provided by the Red Cross as a 'comfort', were rolled with great dexterity. The boys remember the common sight of men with a wad of tobacco in the palm of one hand, using the heel of the other hand to knead the tobacco into shape. Then, in a few seconds, often one-handed, it was rolled, wrapped in paper, licked wet, sealed and you had your cigarette: a slick operation. Then a wax Vesta match would be conjured, struck on a trouser leg and the smoking would start. The soon-soggy tip sat on lips everywhere. In no time a couple of hundred roaming chimney stacks moved about the asylum.

———

The best time of all with the patients—and the highlight of the boys' week—was undoubtedly the weekly Red Cross concert. Nothing was so anticipated, or widened their young eyes or set their pulses pounding as much as this.

Every Sunday the boys raced up the gravel road outside their house towards the water tower, which stood at the apex of the hill. About halfway up the hill was the wooden hall where the concerts were held. David remembers that he and Jack were always smartly clad (something their mother insisted upon), wearing polished black shoes, long socks and short pants. At the hall's entrance the two boys milled about with the hundred or so patients lathering about them, all edging forward to get the best seats.

At the entrance were posters advertising upcoming movies, 'usually a Western that had finished its run in town'. When the door was flung open, Jack and David dashed to their favourite spot— the front row—followed by scores of patients, filling the hall to the brim within minutes.

The hall was typical of its time, and remains a bit of blur to the boys: there were timber floors, and individual wooden chairs were set in rows, with benches at the back. At the front, the stage rose to their shoulders and on it was an upright piano.

The afternoon always started with the playing of 'God Save the King', and all stood, erect and respectful. It is interesting to observe how even the most disturbed psychiatric patient, when placed in a social situation where a certain behaviour is expected can, momentarily, conform to the task. How some manic patients stilled themselves sufficiently, or the occasional depressed patients found the vitality to rise from their chairs, remains a mystery.

The Sunday concert could include a movie or a magician or a musician, and sometimes a puppet show. David remembers how the audience responded:

The patients would roar their approval and stamp their feet. Punch and Judy was a highlight for us. The patients loved it. The patients all loved the songs and they all joined in, many of the patients played music themselves, most of them seemed to be able to whistle a tune; commonly patients played a mouth organ, a small one, often kept in their pocket, or they played a kazoo around the grounds, or played a comb; they always had a comb in their pockets, usually their top outside jacket pocket; and would wrap a piece of tissue paper around the comb and put it against their mouth and play.

Someone would sing on stage, usually with a piano accordion. Lots of Irish songs, Jack and I would remember the words to this day to the songs because they sang the same ones so often: 'When Irish eyes are smiling', 'Molly Malone', 'On the Road to Gundagai' and 'Botany Bay', 'Click Go the Shears' and all the war songs. Vera Lynn was a favourite: 'White Cliffs of Dover', 'We'll Meet Again'. All the men would sing and roar approval.

The men stomped their boots hard upon the reverberating timbers and roared and laughed and sang for the afternoon, the same songs each week. Some were songs of remembrance; some were anthems of defiance—directed towards a hated wartime enemy. The 'Colonel Bogey March' was the classic whistling song for the patients and they'd sit upright and whistle this again and again.

At the concert's conclusion, the door opened, letting a narrow shaft of light into the dark interior. The two boys and the hundred or so patients flowed out through this slit in the wall, a thin stream pouring down the hill—a few patients still marching in time and whistling 'Colonel Bogey' all the way back to their wards.

Virtually all the patients, it seemed to the boys, owned a pocket knife and whittled away on pine bark; pine trees were plentiful on the grounds. Like sailors working on whale bone on long sea-voyages, the patients worked on what was at hand, and it seems as if the pocket knives were of no concern to the medical and nursing staff; certainly the boys never felt alarmed. In their exceptionally generous way, the men gave presents to the boys, one being beautiful carved wooden boats: 'They carved the bark; the toy boats were magnificent,' says David. 'Jack and I had one, mine was called the "Lady Harriet", and the masts were almost a metre high with full rigging; it was beautifully carved and would actually sail.'

The patients also taught the boys how to set rabbit traps. These heavy metallic traps had huge claws, with interlocking teeth, like some lurking deep-sea monster. How the patients had access to such lethal instruments the boys cannot recall, but the obvious fact that such an apparatus might be a danger in the hands of a patient seemed of little concern to the boys. They simply saw adventure. The claws of these traps were 'about the size of our fingers' and, opened up flat, the traps were buried in loose dirt. 'The patients showed us how to operate them, and where to put them in the paddocks. They showed us where the rabbit runs were, near the creek.'

The boys weren't the only ones interested in hunting rabbits. There were no houses for miles into the distance around the Bundoora Mental Hospital, and the paddocks that stretched westward as far as the boys could see, were stuffed with rabbits. That appealed to the boys and also to their father, for Dr John Cade was a shooter with a sharp eye. 'Dad had an old Winchester single shot pea rifle, he'd had it since he was a kid.'

When John returned from the wards, late in the afternoon, without any suggestion of changing from his coat and tie, he would set out from home, gun slung over shoulder, step over the gravel road, slip through the barbed-wire fence and head down to the creek, whose course could be seen from afar, running alongside the spiny thicket of blackberry bushes. The boys would follow eagerly.

When the trio of hunters returned later in the evening, the shooting doctor and his two small boys came back as they'd left, dumping the rifle, bullets and quarry—usually rabbits, but sometimes a hare—in the laundry. John then set to skinning and gutting. He was good at this, and his hands moved fast, precisely. Unruffled, and still in his work clothes, he soon had the stringy meat of a carcass. Sometimes he would wrap the carcass in a hessian bag, to ward off flies, and hang it in the laundry until it ripened, slowly, ready for eating. He loved jugged hare, that somewhat anachronistic gamey English dish. One culinary tradition entailed braising the hare slowly in its own juices and blood, with a touch of red wine and a handful of berries. The stench—blood of hare and gut of rabbit—that drifted from the young doctor's house must have aroused the curiosity of patients and attendants. But none of that mattered to John. He did what he wanted to do regardless of the enquiring looks of those around him.

12

An idea smouldered in John's broad-gauge mind. It had, even before Changi, but Changi made it glow. It was an idea that came, not from any psychiatric line of thought, but from a study of food and nutrition, and how the smallest of elements affected people's bodies and minds. And there is evidence, from John's library, of how that idea came about.

John Cade was a prodigious reader of books. Fortunately for us, he was of that school of readers who jot their impressions in the margins as they read. Equally fortunately, some of his library remains, with his characteristic, precise notations and his immaculate underlining. In these jottings he has left us clues as to what he did during those critical years from 1946—clues that require some deciphering but they are an aperture into his mind.

On the inside cover of his books, John, characteristically, wrote his name and date of purchase—we wouldn't expect anything else from this punctilious man. So we know that in the year he started his classic experiments, 1946, he purchased a book, *Recent Advances in Endocrinology*—hardly a title to turn heads. The author was a certain A.T. Cameron, a controversial British-born Canadian Professor of Biochemistry, who wrote about the body's hormones and not really anything much at all about mental health. We might think this unusual reading for a psychiatrist, but it almost certainly reflected John's view that he was first a physician, and second, a psychiatrist. It was a private joke among colleagues that he rarely went anywhere without a stethoscope stuffed into his coat pocket. John Cade, the doctor, saw the body and brain as a chemical laboratory.

The first organ discussed by Professor Cameron—the thyroid gland—was of keen interest to John, and he underlined in immaculate blue fountain pen ink all that fascinated him. It set him on a clear path. Cade was intrigued by how the thyroid gland—a butterfly-shaped organ that sits at the front of the neck—could alter behaviour. When it is overactive, the thyroid gland secretes excessive amounts of hormones, powerful substances capable of triggering changes elsewhere in the body. In response, the body rocks in agitation and the mind is flung into restless thought. When, however, the thyroid gland is underactive, less of the hormones are secreted and the body is sluggish and the mind impoverished. It was a model that had a profound impact on the way John thought about one particular psychiatric illness: manic depression.

John speculated: was it possible that an excess of some unknown chemical orbiting your body made you manic—with all its wild elevation—and, if so, then maybe a deficiency of this same chemical made you depressed? It was a simple notion: excess of something in the body caused mania; deficiency caused depression. It was this slip of an idea that set him on a pathway of discovery.

Manic-depressive illness had long intrigued John. If anything, it was the black depressions of the illness that moved him the most.

Jean recalled a remark typical of her husband:

> If you saw some of those melancholics it would break your heart. They just sit in the airing court and don't do anything. They might just pick their fingernails. If I could just get them out of themselves . . .

So in 1946, John's starting point was a belief that mania was caused by an excess of a naturally occurring substance in the body, a type of intoxication if you like. And that depression was the opposite— a deficiency of this naturally occurring substance. Now of course, all this was wild speculation because he certainly had no idea if such a substance existed in the body and, even if it did, he had even less idea of how to find it. Still, this was his launching point.

John Cade was a pragmatic man. The practical question he had to answer was this: how could he possibly know what was happening inside the manic-depressive brains of the men for whom he cared? There were no modern imaging devices to chart the structure and size of the brain in 1946. Repeated blood tests were intrusive and, anyhow, none were known to point to any specific type of mental disorder. What could John examine in order to find this imagined substance that caused mania in excess? His answer, perhaps surprisingly, was urine.

Jean remembers the start of her husband's experiments: 'He came to me and said: "I've got to do some research on why these patients have got different illnesses. I'd like to find the melancholias first. I've got an idea that might come to something if I save a lot of jars.' Why her husband needed jars for this work was not immediately apparent to her, but soon the jars started accumulating.

John travelled to the city and purchased numerous bulky glass jars from McEwans, a department store in Melbourne. His wife, seeing her house, then garage, bulge with these jars, was less enthusiastic. 'We had no money, I kept telling him.' But John, on a determined line of thinking, was oblivious to his wife's concerns.

'I was horrified, we couldn't afford it. He just said: "we might be able to use them afterwards for pickles".' This, undoubtedly, was a private joke of John's, for as soon as he had acquired sufficient numbers of jars, John started to fill them with urine from his patients. To examine the urine of his patients might seem bizarre to us but it would not have seemed the least bit odd to John Cade. Doctors had long considered urine to be the portal into a man's body and mind.

To the average person, urine is hardly worth more than a passing—if sly and mildly distasteful—look. Whatever anyone else might think of urine, it was about to receive John's complete attention. It was an examination of urine that led him to a series of experiments that would change the course of medical history.

John's thinking ran like this: if mania was due to an excess of a chemical circulating in the body, then just maybe some of this excess chemical might be expelled in the urine. What he was hoping to find was an excess of this putative chemical in the urine of manic patients. If he could prove this, then, it might set him on a path to find a treatment for mania.

He hit upon the idea of comparing urine from patients with different illnesses. Did the urine of a manic-depressive man differ from that of a man with schizophrenia, he wondered. John instructed the ward attendants to place a metal container at the foot of each man's bed. Each morning melancholics, manics and schizophrenics—the tribes of men whose afflictions had rendered the Bundoora asylum their home—were requested, reminded, perhaps cajoled into emptying their bladders into these metal repositories. It was asylum lore that early morning urine was the most potent brew to collect, any chemicals being concentrated overnight. If anything was to be found, it would be found there.

When it came to the art and science of collecting urine, the nursing staff found all they needed to know in their 'red bible', the *Handbook for Mental Nurses*. They cradled this book, thumbed it and flicked through its pages. It highlighted routine, rigidity and responsibility: the triad of asylum life. And nothing was more written up, measured or indicative of this world of fixed habits than the collection of urine.

Once collected, each patient's urine was emptied into one of John's glass jars. Inquisitive medical minds had for centuries pored over the significance of urine taken from patients with every type of illness—mental or otherwise. The hues of urine, they speculated, might reflect the mood of the patient, and doctors for years had scribbled descriptions of this liquid, like vignerons rapturously hanging words in the air about a vintage year.

We can imagine John picking up one of the dozens of glass jars of urine and placing it before the light, examining what could be examined—colour, density, turbidity—looking for the secrets sealed within that might reflect the minds of the men for whom he cared. What John did each day, as he lifted these bottles to the sunlight, was the timeless act of the medical investigator.

John had no laboratory so he started work in his garage in the backyard—not the first or last time something revolutionary in the world of science would miraculously unfold in a garage. The jars accumulated, filling the shelves while he searched for a laboratory. As it turned out, there was one literally less than a hundred metres away over the back fence; an empty pantry in a new ward just built but as yet unoccupied. Jean remembers the day he proudly showed her his find: 'He helped himself to the pantry of this new ward. He took me over to look at it: "Look, look I have a bench and hot and cold water", everything he needed. And so it began from there.'

Everyone called this make-shift laboratory, 'the shed'. The shed—in the timeless tradition of Australian men—was where John kept the tools of trade for his experiments. To get to the shed from the Cade house was a short stroll: out through the gate in the back fence, past the chook pen with its Australorps and Rhode Island Reds, along the gravel path that John took every day. To the right was the paddock with Betty and Kate, grazing and dozing, as draft horses must—then the path continued to the wire door of 'the shed'.

John was just about ready to start his experiments, but he needed one further vital piece of equipment—something cold in which to store and preserve his ever-increasing number of jars of urine.

In a decision that horrified his wife, but seemed natural to John, he chose to store the bottles of urine in the refrigerator in the kitchen of his house. The Cade fridge, with its creamy, rounded shoulders, was a Frigidaire model—an Australian post-war symbol of middle-class wealth; *The Australian Women's Weekly* beamed advertisements displaying the modern fridge's exceptional capacity to keep fresh and cool home-made jams, butter and beer. The importance of keeping urine chilled seemed to have escaped the magazine editors. None of this impressed Jean, but her protests failed to deter her husband; utility always trumped fashion. Each patient's urine was decanted into a screw-top bottle, numbered and shelved. Beneath the butter sat the urine of dozens of patients: amber brews drawn from mute and immobile melancholic men; fizzing brews from over-the-top manic men that needed a baker's dozen of nurses to pin down. Every time anyone from the Cade family opened the Frigidaire door, there, staring at them, were the bodily fluids of several dozen mentally ill men.

For the two boys, it was perfectly natural to push aside a bottle or two of urine to find the cheese, all done with the casualness of childhood. 'To us it was all normal. We wouldn't have known whether everybody else did or didn't have urine in their fridges at home.'

John Cade set about storing the urine of mentally ill men in the household fridge with no quiver of doubt, and with a single-mindedness that his wife struggled to accept but finally, resistance whittled away, simply did. And with that, the bottles of urine proliferated to fill whatever chilled cavity remained in this household that ran to a very different tune.

John, almost comically, had glass jars full of urine multiplying and accumulating. Now what to do with them? Well, he did something we might consider cruel, but was natural to an experimentally minded doctor with a hunch. He had no sophisticated equipment to analyse urine, even if he knew what he was looking for. Crude and simple, with shades of Dr Moreau, he decided to inject the urine he had collected into guinea pigs to see how the urine might affect the animals.

Sometime in 1946, John obtained guinea pigs from nearby Mont Park asylum and caged them in his newly acquired 'laboratory'. His second son David still treasures the memory of walking into the pantry and seeing his father with the guinea pigs:

The guinea pigs were in cages, but we also had some at home. They got through a lot of kitchen scraps. I remember Dad handling one of them on his left arm, and stroking it; they were tame from constant handling. They were good-looking: tan, black and white. My favourite was a tan and brown one.

Jean adds: 'We had guinea pigs in the shed. Lots of guinea pigs. As they died we'd get some more. He was good to them. He'd call them darling. And say: "Don't you mind me doing this" as he injected them.'

John would draw urine from the stored jars into a syringe. The syringes were not the lightweight plastic jobs of today. They were hefty and industrial in design, constructed of glass and metal. They clanged and scraped when assembled, and when sterilised in pots. He would gently hold and turn over the guinea pigs, and inject the urine into their abdominal cavities. It takes little to imagine him moving assuredly and with celerity from jar of urine to syringe to animal.

John was looking to see if urine from a manic patient might affect a guinea pig differently to urine from other patients. One by one, regardless of the diagnosis of the patient, the guinea pigs perished. And, practising what he'd done all his professional life, and what any respectable doctor might do, he performed a post-mortem on every animal, looking for a deeper understanding of what caused mental illness.

As the guinea pigs died, he procured more animals and started afresh. Each evening after work and when he had time during the day, he returned to this pantry and worked alone with his animals.

John was well aware that what he was doing was remarkably crude. So, at first, he kept quiet about his work, telling only a select few who needed to know. Those in the loop included the head of Victoria's mental health services, Dr John Catarinich, a family friend of the Cades, who organised payment for all the chemicals John used. Today, no one would consider whipping out, buying dozens of jars, filling them with the urine of patients and then injecting the urine into guinea pigs. It sounds archaic and primitive, and it was an era of experimental crudity that was coming to an end. But somehow his upbringing, his pragmatism and his insatiable curiosity gave rise to this hands-on experimentation; it had been the shaping of a lifetime that led him here.

Although in these early days, John kept knowledge of his experiments close to his chest, even the most solitary of workers craves some recognition or, at least, someone with whom they can discuss their hopes and anxieties about their work. John's quest was something he wanted to share with another person, someone who might appreciate his endeavours. He turned to his father.

John Cade's father could be unapproachable and cold, more so as he grew older. His time in Gallipoli had left him wounded in the way of so many men: irritable, impatient, and drifting into depression. With an attraction to bombast, some called him a snob, or, if polite, pedantic. Nevertheless, John bundled up his ideas and made a path to his father. But it was always going to be a formidable task.

When John and Jean arrived at David Cade's home they typically ended up in the lounge, sitting in armchairs near the fireplace. John, as he'd done as a boy, continued to address his father as 'sir'. If John anticipated curiosity and warmth, he was to be disappointed; David Cade was not open to his son's scientific ideas, and grew impatient almost from the start. Fustily attired in a three-piece suit, David Cade Snr was light on humour and bamboozled by the chemistry his son spouted. His father—more at home with a style of medicine closer to the nineteenth century than the mid-twentieth—was relieved when he diverted his son from scientific discussions.

John's son David, in recalling these conversations, described his grandfather:

> He'd sit in his armchair with his elbows on the arms of the chair and his fingertips together in front of his face . . . Dad would be standing in front of the fireplace with his back to the mantelpiece and you knew it wouldn't be long before Grandpa started saying 'Yes, yes . . . John' He never gave Dad long to explain his ideas . . . he'd say 'Look, you know I'm not a scientific man, I'm a classical scholar' and he'd talk over Dad at times.

Jack also recalled that his grandfather chopped the conversations with 'yes, yes' and moved on, suggesting either a lack of understanding or interest or both.

John took the cold indifference of his father poorly and complained bitterly to Jean of his father's lack of interest: 'I don't know why I care . . . Dad's not interested in anything I do.'

John returned to injecting, observing and performing post-mortems on the rapidly increasing number of dead guinea pigs. When he returned from his afternoon rounds he made straight for his laboratory. Jean remembers how intense, how frustrated her husband became at this time: 'He didn't tell me. He didn't tell anyone of us what he was doing. He wanted to work all by himself. He wanted no interruptions at all.'

His isolation in his shed, in some ways, was a benefit, and gave him great latitude to trust his instincts and pursue any and every unexpected finding to his satisfaction. Jean said of him that he was sometimes a dreamer and 'liked to follow his own thoughts through and branch off on to other things' without hindrance.

This was a time of intense concentration and longing for John, driven as he was to find some meaning in the experiments he was conducting. With uncompromising single-mindedness, he ransacked his mind for ideas and kept fiddling with combinations and injecting guinea pigs.

This bleak period of sustained experimental work presaged something much darker in the final days of winter—something John could not have foreseen.

————

When John returned from war, like many men, he reflected on the time lost. He felt an urgency to make up for this vacuum. Jean explained: 'When he returned John wanted more children, feeling he'd missed out on the first two boys.' John was keen to start, and felt the press of time.

Jean gave birth to a baby girl, Mary, on 25 August 1946. She lived only 24 hours. The pregnancy had been smooth, as far as pregnancies go, and Mary was full term: a normal child was expected. At least this is how Jean remembers it. The family memory is that Mary was squeezed empty of blood by her mother's abnormally contracting womb, accidentally and tragically, and was born white and floppy. The death certificate indicates that the cause of death was 'erythroblastosis foetalis', an incompatability between the mother's blood and the baby's blood, leading to anaemia. As was the custom of the time, Jean Cade was forbidden to see her dead daughter, but over 50 years later wistfully remembered: 'I was just told she looked like a little angel.'

It was left to John to organise Mary's funeral.

The two boys didn't go to their sister's funeral at nearby Heidelberg Cemetery, 'but we heard from our uncle that it was a tiny funeral and that Dad carried the coffin in one hand'. John once wrote that carrying his dead daughter, in her small white coffin, was the saddest moment of his life. He never spoke about Mary to his boys or about their shared loss.

John rarely displayed unrestrained emotions in public; men of the time behaved this way. But Changi had also seen to it that when a swell of emotion threatened his equilibrium, such emotion was clipped hard. Nothing wasteful, even emotion, was allowed. Some who met him for the first time after the war recall a self-contained and slightly remote man.

After the funeral John returned to his experiments. He stepped back into a private world: a pantry filled with guinea pigs, syringes and a wealth of urine. In here, he need not dwell upon the death of his daughter, or at least, he might try to submerge what grief and bitterness he felt, so that those around him could only see what they'd always seen: the undemonstrative Dr Cade, who did what he had to do.

13

Suburban Bundoora is not what it used to be. If you are looking for a sense of place or a sense of history on the old hospital grounds where John worked, you might struggle. Above the line of eucalypts, a KFC sign, brash and plastic, is visible; it is hard to re-imagine the world of the late 1940s with such a gaudy neon emblem intruding.

Bundoora Mental Hospital no longer exists. Dismantled in 1993, only a few remnant buildings, like members of a near-extinct species, have managed to hold out. John's 'shed' is gone; Jack Cade, the oldest son, can still point to where it stood. We know this for sure because Jack took a series of photographs in 1980, in an effort to save the shed as a heritage site. In one photo the shed is framed at the top by a large overarching bough of a massive gum tree. Today, the tree's girth has expanded a little but its distinctive arching shape and signature markings are identifiable. When we stand next to this tree, we stand before the shed as it was in 1946. The gum tree remains as a silent historical witness to John's work.

The photos also take us inside the shed, which is immediately recognisable to Jack—unchanged from the 1940s. Cupboards line the floor on one side of the room; above them a bench and a sink, where John conducted his guinea pig experiments. Above the sink are heavy timbered sash windows.

We walk towards where the Cade family house stood—that's gone as well. Jack points out another two gum trees that stood just outside the back fence of their house. The trees mark the direction in which John struck out each day from home to the wards. Today, in the absence of so much that was man-made, the markers that tell us the most are the eucalypts that peg where house and wards once stood. John Cade would have liked that.

———

In 1946 John was a man in a hurry. Later in life he wrote: 'I returned from three and a half years as a POW of the Japanese mourning the wasted years and determined to pursue the ideas that had germinated in that interminable time.'

These few lines suggest that Changi had been a kind of crucible for John, in which to think about his notions of mental illness. Unhelpfully, though, John never expanded on what ideas did take root during his time as a POW, but clearly something creative strained within him.

John was a self-described 'lone wolf' researcher who preferred to labour on his own. He did not seek out a mentor to foster those tingles of imaginative thought or, until years later, supervise research students. And he was no chemist, but he had knowledge gleaned from Changi and, as part of his work at Bundoora, he routinely prepared prescription medications for his patients, often from the basic chemicals.

John pursued a number of leads over the next eighteen months. His early experiments suggested to him that the urine from manic patients was more toxic than urine from other patients, and therefore killed more guinea pigs. As it turns out, John's belief that manic urine was more toxic was false—urine from a manic patient is no more likely to kill a guinea pig than any other sort of urine. This mistake, like countless others that scientists have made over the centuries, was a fortunate one, as it spurred him on, and he continued unhindered with his idiosyncratic research.

John's mind bubbled in anticipation of finding something in the urine of manic patients. What could it be? There are two known toxic substances in urine—urea and uric acid. Both are breakdown products, halfway houses of the body's metabolism. Perhaps one of them was the elusive chemical toxin he was after.

Some of John's chemical experiments make for intriguing reading. Left for posterity, they resemble the scribbles one might find in a high school chemistry notebook. At one point he adds 3 cubic centimetres of hydrochloric acid to every 100 cubic centimetres of urine to get a precipitate and then he takes us through the steps of filtering; there is more than a whiff of a home economics class when John writes that he adds 'one level teaspoon' of charcoal for every 100 cc. And then, when he reminds himself to 'shake for 5–10 minutes', he appears in our minds, absurdly, behind a cocktail bar as if preparing an evening gin and tonic.

When finally done, John hit upon the idea that urea was the toxic element in all the urines that killed the guinea pigs. The conclusion he drew was that there was more urea in manic urine than in the urine of patients with other mental conditions. But when he tested this idea he found that manic urine had no more urea than any other urine. He was stuck.

To get over this setback he postulated that urea and uric acid might work in tandem to make the urine of manic patients more toxic.

He started to work on uric acid, and this is where his experiments grew fascinating. To make up different strengths of uric acid he needed to convert it into a substance that he could more easily manipulate. On its own, uric acid would not dissolve in water. To persuade it to do so, John added the element lithium to uric acid to make up a compound called lithium urate. And that is where lithium comes onto the scene, *en passant*, almost apologetically.

In the course of trying different combinations, as any good scientist might, John then injected lithium alone, as lithium carbonate solution. That's when he drew breath, and promptly forgot everything else, except for lithium.

When John injected the lithium, the guinea pigs seemed restful. In one memorable description he said that he simply lifted one of the guinea pigs, turned it over, and placed it gently on its back. Instead of doing what any respectable guinea pig should do when placed in such a vulnerable position—turn over and stand up in protest—this guinea pig simply lay on its back and looked vacantly at John. He repeated this experiment again, and the response was the same.

Behind John's unfathomable face something stirred, a shaft of comprehension.

Uncharacteristically agitated, he summoned his wife, a day she remembered. 'He called me from the kitchen, with great excitement, to come and see.' And John showed Jean how, without any difficulty, he could turn a guinea pig over on to its back and move it around without any protest. These lovable rodents, normally a mass of vibrating muscle and fur, now with lithium in their bellies, would lie with equanimity on their backs, staring with soft eyes at John while he gently prodded them with the stub of his index finger. He had never seen them behave like this. They seemed alert, but they were calm.

So what was going on here? John thought that the lithium was calming the rodents. Looking back, it is more likely that the guinea pigs were ill, due to the toxic effects of an excessive dose of lithium. But John didn't know this. What he saw was a rodent stilled by lithium.

There are times, when reading John's carefully written accounts of his experiments, that it is virtually impossible to follow his line of thinking. He was wrong when he concluded that urine from manic patients was more toxic than other urine. He was also probably wrong when he thought the guinea pigs were resting after lithium. Many of his observations cannot be replicated when tried today, so reproducibility, the gold standard for scientific sturdiness, is absent. But none of this mattered. Because when John nimbly sifted through the options, his mind intuited something remarkable: that giving lithium to guinea pigs soothed them in a way that was worth pursuing. There was something special about lithium.

But where did lithium come from, and what did anyone really know about it?

14

Lithium, from the Greek *lithos* meaning stone, is, aptly, dug from the earth. Discovered in 1817, any high school chemistry student will know its place in the Periodic Table—the lightest and most reactive of all metals. So light is it, that this soft silvery metal floats on water. Lithium has been around from the very beginnings of the universe—at the Big Bang only three elements were fused in that furnace: hydrogen, helium and lithium. It is found and used in the most astonishing variety of places—everyone knows about lithium batteries, but probably not that lithium is a lethal component of the hydrogen bomb. When you gaze upwards on New Year's Eve and marvel at the incandescent pyrotechnics and the night sky turning blood-crimson, you are gazing at lithium burning in the heavens.

Lithium is a bewitching element and, when in the form of lithium chloride powder, absorbs moisture from the air and melts before your eyes. But what would John have known about lithium, alone in his shed, tinkering with his chemical concoctions?

To find a clue to that question, we can start with the 1947 *Australian and New Zealand Pharmaceutical Formulary*. This was the drug manual available to young doctors in Australia. It is a book steeped in apothecary lore. Its powders and brews are balanced on beams, and measured in terms carved from antiquity—grains for mass and minims for volume. On page 55, typical of this craft, we find the mystical ingredients of rhubarb powder; and of syrup of ginger; and of a tincture of cudbear, whatever that may be (apparently a colouring obtainable from certain lichens). And as for lithium? Well, there is nothing. Not on page 55, nor on any other page.

But if we turn back just six years to Martindale's *Extra Pharmacopoeia* of 1941 (22nd edition) or further back to a classic of the genre, Squire's *Companion to the British Pharmacopoeia* of 1916, that's where lithium finds its form. In the latter there are no less than ten densely packed pages dedicated to the healing powers of lithium. And it is here that the well-known forms of medicinal lithium are laid out for the reader—lithium carbonate, lithium citrate and lithium chloride. In these older hospital texts John Cade would have found plenty on lithium, but only a little to advance his thinking.

To understand how lithium entered medicine we have to go back to the mid-nineteenth century when it was introduced for the treatment of gout. Indeed some of its proponents suggested that recurrent gout could cause mania and melancholia, and that lithium might heal these states. Then, in 1871, American military physician and neurologist William Hammond reported using lithium bromide in the treatment of mania. But nothing further came from it. Around the same time, two Danish doctors, Carl Lange and his brother, Fritz, treated recurring depression with lithium but publication of their work in Danish and German restricted their audience and their approach fell into disuse. John Cade, it seems, was completely unaware of these early endeavours to use lithium in psychiatric illness.

By the late 1940s, notions of lithium's supposed curative properties in all diseases had lost favour and it seems to be included in reference books, almost apologetically, as a testament to past faulty medical thinking. But importantly the doses used for the various lithium preparations were noted: something that John would need.

Although in the late nineteenth century, lithium was mistakenly heralded as a treatment for gout, it did propel lithium into homes and hospitals around the world. And when it was found to be present in natural spring waters, lithium was celebrated as part of a water cure. In Squire's *Companion* of 1916, no less than fourteen pages are devoted to the healing claims of spa waters around the globe: in Baden-Baden, Germany, 'The Lithia Waters contain about 3 grains of lithium chloride in 20 oz ... For rheumatoid arthritis, chronic gouty affections and paralysis'. In another spa in Germany it was held to 'stimulate the intestines and urinary organs' and the Bavarians found it wonderfully congenial for managing 'haemorrhoids and constipation'. In the drawing rooms of medical establishments in England and Wales, lithium waters held hope for those afflicted with 'hepatic and intestinal congestion, gastric affections, for gouty and rheumatic affections, diabetes, eczema, kidney troubles'. Nothing, it seemed, was too much for the all-curative power of lithium. People flocked to the waters and lithium soon found a favoured place in popular culture.

It was almost inevitable, therefore, that lithium's supposed power of restoration would also find a home in fiction. And it did.

H.G. Wells, grandmaster of science-fiction writing, could have used the soothing power of lithium waters in his own turbulent life. Whether he did we don't know, but he found a use for it in his writing.

Lithium, and its calming powers entered at a crucial point in his 1895 short story 'The Reconciliation', which told of two men— Temple and Findlay—once the warmest of friends but now the most bitter of enemies. As lithium is swallowed, momentarily an old friendship returns:

> 'There's no woman worth a man's friendship,' said Temple abruptly. He sat down in an easy chair, poured out and drank a dose of whisky and lithia. The idea of friendship took possession of him, and he became reminiscent of student days and student adventures. For some time it was, 'Do you remember' this, and 'Do you remember' that. And Findlay grew cheerful again.

In this story, the two men meet after a prolonged separation, but as they continue to talk, spiteful memories are rekindled and resentment festers. The men, both intellectuals and scientists, wrangle with their own bestial emotions. They struggle to quell violent desires to hurt one another. As the memory of their dispute over a woman surfaces, civility cracks. Temple, drinking to excess, warmed his cheeks to a fighting red.

Lithium water stirred with whisky was a gentleman's drink in H.G. Wells' tale, a balm to settle unsteady heads—although perhaps not a balm of sufficient strength. For as the drama concludes, the whisky clouds their humanity and, like the savages within that they sought to conceal, they brawl viciously until Temple crushes the skull of his one-time friend.

If nothing else, Wells' story of these two men suggests the drinking of lithium as a restorative was seen to be natural and available to a nineteenth-century English gentleman. But John Cade's life was lived beyond the rim of such fiction. Lithium had assumed a place in late-nineteenth-century English life that was vastly different to the post-war Melbourne that John inhabited. In the late 1940s lithium was not only absent in Australian popular culture, it was barely mentioned within the medical world.

It has always been a mystery as to where John found his lithium. Sadly, he never commented on this, and we are left dangling and guessing. It is possible that different preparations of lithium were stored in hospitals, remnants from the end of the nineteenth century and early twentieth century, stockpiled in the backrooms and dispensaries—overlooked and unused. If one stumbled into an asylum dispensary in the 1940s, one stepped into a world of the past, and along the rows of deep-brown medicinal jars you might have found some filled with lithium powders. Relics from the heyday of lithium, they stood as silent witness to earlier medical theory when John Cade made the decision to resurrect them for his experiments. Or perhaps John sought lithium from a drug house;

we don't know. In the end he had enough lithium to continue his work.

In lithium, John had something tangible to work with, but his notes reveal that it was not only lithium that attracted his notice. During his experiments, at different times John tried just about every element he could lay his hands on: calcium, magnesium, titanium, rubidium, beryllium, cobalt, nickel, zinc, tungsten, molybdenum, selenium. A who's who of the Periodic Table. But, in the end, only lithium worked.

His years in Changi offered John a different view of life: that you take your chances, knowing that they will, as all life will, run dry. That you have to work out pretty quickly what's important and what's not, and that bunkum and squandering of time is not to be tolerated.

John Cade's observation, that lithium soothed guinea pigs, was intriguing but it could have remained just the stump of an idea. It took a decisive act—courageous and maybe even a little reckless—to make something of that moment.

15

In the weeks leading up to March 1948, John Cade did something that was unexpected, secretive. Not shameful, as his cryptic act might suggest, but certainly an action he wished no one to observe, much less challenge him about.

He resolved to test lithium on himself, before giving it to his patients.

To a naive eye, this might seem daring, boldness bequeathed to few. Or perhaps it was just ill-considered, or foolish. If he wanted someone to experiment on, why didn't he just give the solution to the first patient he thought suitable?

The answer, most likely, lay in John's character.

John Cade in 1948 was a blend of the military and the medical; it was never likely that he would inflict an untried potion on an innocent man until he had weathered its effects himself. For a man who had survived three and a half years' incarceration as a POW, the act of self-experimentation and a preparedness to take chances had become a way of life.

Of course, no mortal eye will ever know what stream of thought pushed John over that line to test lithium on himself, but the stakes were high: 1948 was a peak year for deaths in Melbourne asylums. In one asylum alone, Royal Park, John recorded in that year there were '183 deaths—that's three and a half a week'. He kept a death tally, recording that two in every fifteen admissions, like the victims of a plague, ended up as a cold slab of flesh.

What we do know is that, strangely, for a man who documented with Swiss precision each injection into his experimental guinea pigs, John left no written vestige of the experiments upon himself. Perhaps this reflected the secretive nature of his act; or awareness of his eccentricity; or of his terror of things going terribly wrong. And of course there was the fear of exposure to ridicule. He knew that, almost certainly, those about him—his psychiatric colleagues, his wife, his father—would frown in disapproval. Some of his colleagues, especially, would smirk if he stumbled; it would confirm that the 'mad major' of Changi was loopy indeed. But John had enough sense of self-preservation to know he'd only be considered loopy if caught.

All John knew for sure was that lithium had led his guinea pigs to lie vacant-eyed and dreamily insensitive to the prodding of human fingers.

As John prepared to take lithium, the spirit of the alchemist stirred within, knowing he was doing what many would regard as against the natural order. He emptied the lithium powder into a test tube, stirred a solution and raised the transparent fluid to his lips. Whatever the nature of the force that guided his hand, it was deep-rooted and arcane.

He held the elixir to his lips: his nostrils sensed no odour, and, with the courage and recklessness anything truly original must embrace, he opened his mouth.

Eyes closed, he drank.

At first, the taste was probably a little salty, almost metallic—something to note for how a patient might react. And then, nothing. Pleasingly, nothing. No collapsing to the floor, no maniacal convulsions, no agonising clutching of body parts about which—in a more hesitant moment—he may have fantasised. Nothing happened; wonderfully, nothing. He cleansed the vial of the solution and put it back on the rack. The world, for the moment, remained as it had five minutes earlier, with equanimity undisturbed.

The following day John returned and did the same. And the next. Each day he returned and subjected his body to whatever his God and the Periodic Table would deal him.

As the clear liquid drained from the glass and into his body, he could only have imagined its course. The mechanic in him knew that the liquid would descend from mouth to oesophagus, and that it would be absorbed, rapidly, all along his gut. The writings from the nineteenth century, familiar to John, suggested that lithium would seek out every organ, seeping into every cell and across the blood–brain barrier, that Great Wall of China, which separated the brain from blood. And it was the brain that was lithium's final target.

As a sophisticated voyeur of the natural world, John now observed his own body and felt its perturbations. It is hard to know what he expected when he felt the liquid upon his tongue, but apart from an involuntary grimace as he experienced its elemental tang and the gurgling of his tummy in faint dispute, he remained well over the next few days. He knew that he must, by logical extension, trial lithium on a patient.

There was, however, one final matter to resolve before he could try out his lithium potion on the diggers about him: telling his wife.

All marriages are a journey of trust, of its observance and of its breaking. And for John Cade, as any good Catholic knew, confession was a cleansing force. He felt compelled to spill the news to Jean that he had ingested lithium for days on end. Years afterwards, she recorded how her fury flickered into a full flame after hearing his confession; how her anger rose from anxiety about losing a husband and a father from reckless experimentation. Whether such marital friction was ever more than a moment's distraction in what he planned next, John does not record. But seemingly without flinching or taking a wavering step, he sought out a patient for whom lithium might work its spell.

16

John's keen eye did not have to scour the wards to find prospective patients; a sweeping glance from his backyard saw all that needed to be seen. Manic patients encircled John, and he penned his thoughts on each one:

> An older man of 63 with mania for the last 'two and a quarter years' claimed to those who listened (and most who did not) that he was valued at over 800,000 pounds and was a fearless soldier. At times, when his grandiosity settled, this warrior proclaimed that he might only be valued at a paltry 500,000 pounds.
>
> A younger man, in his 40s, manic for 2 months—strode triumphantly across the asylum grounds, flinging his arms about, gesticulating wildly to those who crossed his path, and bellowed into the night until the sounds dissipated miles beyond the asylum walls. He ate ravenously, when anything was put before him, pouring food into his gob to feed his thin frame and fuel a rampant energy.
>
> One man had been in and out of asylums for 30 years, tormented by the delusion of a wireless tampering with his brain; another ex-soldier communicated only by a form of magical telepathy with those he trusted; and another who,

with elastic ease, ranted for hours on end at the mysteries of a brick wall.

Or there was the young immigrant Polish doctor, now a manic patient at the neighbouring Mont Park asylum, whose buoyant mood compelled him to perform somersaults on admission to the asylum and, when landing upright, flashed a grin and beamed to his psychiatrist that he needed 'intercourse 12 times' every evening to quell his urgent appetite. Cursing his fate, agitated and screaming, he struck another patient, giggling unrepentantly. He was locked in a single room, daubing faeces over the walls.

Other men, though prodigious beings of overwhelming physical power, remained pleasantly elevated, amiable giants. Some manic patients were vagrants, scooped up by police from the streets of Melbourne and unloaded at Bundoora.

But for all their eccentricities, their oddness, and the hazy worlds into which they withdrew, John's writing reflects his fondness for them. Not only were most ex-soldiers—an affinity that cut deeper for him than any other—they were men of a common, decent cut.

As evening set in, and the sun sank behind the hills where the Cade boys had primed their rabbit traps, the wards of the asylum unbolted their heavy timbered doors, inviting in and welcoming for the night all those who wandered the grounds. At day's end, the commotion and the laughter and the crying finally came to a halt— the daily din exhausted. It was then that the manic patients settled in their beds. When the lights went out—and all was still and dark— the only sound heard was the human hum of 200 crackling brains.

Urgency snapped at John's heels: to find, without delay, a patient suitable for his lithium experiment. That sentiment and his need to make up for lost time from the war pressed him towards his goal.

Among the wriggling mass of the mentally ill was one patient whom John knew well: William Brand, more commonly known as Bill or Billy.

It was Bill who he thought might respond to lithium.

17

Bill Brand's embattled story is his own, but it is also a universal one. The struggle to survive with a mental illness on the streets of an unforgiving world scarred him, as did dealing with a brutish bureaucracy that slapped him down whenever he sought a raise in his army pension. It is not a stretch to suggest that his life story is probably the most important in Australian psychiatric history.

Bill arrived in Australia as part of that great heave of Commonwealth migration in the early twentieth century. South African by birth, he entered the world near Cape Town sometime in the mid- to late 1890s. The exact date of his birth is elusive in official records, and, unofficially, Bill's age shifts about; even Bill was never sure of his precise age. The manifest of the *Cycle*—the ship upon which his family arrived in Australia—records Bill as a boy of primary school age when he stepped upon Australian soil in 1907.

Bill had a truncated education—just a handful of years at a state school. Since leaving school at fourteen, he had variously laboured on a farm, learnt carpentry skills, and ridden as a rough-and-ready jockey breaking-in horses.

Early in the First World War, the Brand family was living in Melbourne. Bill's father, a self-taught carpenter, had signed up for service with the Australian Light Horse in 1915, but had already been invalided out. A desperate call went out for young men to volunteer for the armed forces; the nineteen-year-old Bill Brand was one who answered. Not, perhaps, an ideal candidate but at least he would replace his father.

Bill's father was a victim of paralysing malaria on the Gallipoli Peninsula, and suffered concussion. He also had that ubiquitous First World War sickness—shell shock—which seemed to embrace a dozen different diagnoses. He was discarded from the Australian Army, unfit, one month before his son stepped into the Melbourne Town Hall on 7 July 1916 to enlist.

It was a dismal day that dawned on Melbourne, and, in an obscure light, so typical of that southern city in winter, William Henry Brand entered the Town Hall, along with a handful of other men. There was not only a depressed weather pattern upon Melbourne that greasy and miserable July day, but there was a dark mood constricting the city. War news filled the newspapers.

Examined by the army doctor, Bill, fully stretched, stood at a jockey's altitude, five feet five and three-quarter inches, and weighed a smidgeon below a bantamweight at eight stone. A yellowing army file tells us that his swarthy skin was discoloured by a mole, a burn scar and vaccination marks. Later, the Sherlock Holmes in John Cade would have seized on each blemish as a story to unfold from this would-be soldier's past—and it was a more varied and pock-marked past than Bill's scant testimony suggested. He had spent many rough hours as a labourer in a tannery and, kicked by a horse years before, his right knee was rickety. But nothing and no one betrayed its weakness that day.

Bill's body was pored over by his medical reviewer for syphilis, defective intelligence, haemorrhoids and traces of corporal punishment. None were found and he was passed medically fit. At no stage, apparently, was he asked about a history of mental illness.

The official archives suggest that Bill may have attempted to join the Australian Light Horse, like his father, but for reasons unknown was accepted into the infantry.

Atop each page of his army file sits his regimental number, unit and battalion, embedded digits that in later years no mental illness could ablate and, even in moments of madness, came to him with ease:

Private William Brand
Regimental No. 6618
21st Unit of the 7th Battalion

To the army he was always known as William Henry Brand, but everyone called him Bill.

In a few scratchy but revealing lines poking above the parapet, the army dossier records Bill as a 'Driver' (presumably of motor cars) and unmarried, living in the city of Melbourne. He had been neither dismissed 'with disgrace' from the military nor did he admit to any police record, nor was he deemed 'incorrigible or worthless' in the penetrating eyes of Australian law. There was little to distinguish him from the thousands of other working-class men who flocked to the call of mother Britain—except on one point. Bill had already been rejected once as 'unfit for His Majesty's Service' because of his 'weak constitution'. What that meant is never explained and, it would seem, in this hour of dire national need, such doubts were swept aside.

William Henry Brand signed his name on his attestation papers: a gawky 'W' and 'H' suggest a schoolboy's best hand. His writing is clumsy—ungainly curlicues—constructed rather than written, like a student composing his first signature to please a teacher. Bill took his Oath of Enlistment and committed until the end of the war 'unless sooner lawfully discharged, dismissed, or removed'—a prescient phrase.

Bill embarked from Melbourne, along with scores of other troops, on 2 October 1916, aboard the *Nestor*, arriving six weeks later in Plymouth, England.

On board he fell sick, and upon arrival in England he was carted to an isolation hospital in Salisbury. His diagnosis was uncertain. He had two lumbar punctures—thin metal probes inserted into his lower back to siphon off the fluid from around his spinal cord and brain—to confirm a possible diagnosis of meningitis. Diagnosed with the suggestive but ultimately vague label of 'cerebrospinal fever (mild case)', it was reported that Bill 'has periods of permanent excitement . . . lacks comprehension . . . does not remember much at all'. His diagnosis was an enigma to his doctors.

Bill's military dossier continues as a string of brief, punctuated statements; the air of turbulence that pervades his life is unmistakeable.

Three months later he was marched from the hospital to his military base. His right knee—the one kicked by a horse years earlier—swelled with fluid during each forced march until Bill could step no more.

Within days he was readmitted to another military hospital, from which he absconded on a three-day escapade. On return, he—in the perverse language of the army—was 'awarded 72 hours detention' and was forced to cough up five days' pay. Five weeks later he was marched to his depot. Medical probing found him less than 'A' class and—while what distinguished 'A' from 'B' category of human health was never revealed—he was scrutinised closely. By July 1917 Bill, now a serial nuisance within army ranks, created 'a disturbance at about midnight . . . damaging government property four panes of glass valued at 5 shillings'. He was forced to make reparations, and pay back the damage bill. Further hospitalisation and detentions followed.

There is an air of the scruffy, of disrepute, if not quite of the unlawful when one read's Bill's military file. And while his may have been an aberrant, disruptive personality on the loose, it rather has the thrum of an awakening mental illness.

Bill's eight months in England were a mishmash of detentions in various hospitals and army depots; and of disorganised and petty criminal behaviour that saw him packed up and on board a ship heading home to Melbourne by the middle of 1917. As Bill prepared to voyage back to Australia, his medical attendant, in a statement not reassuring to the crew, warned: 'This man is suffering from dementia and should be under control.' Whatever medical diagnosis afflicted him, Bill's mind was unleashed and beyond understanding.

Not a great deal is recorded of Bill's wayward return voyage but clearly it was not without its problems. The swelling about his knee subsided and he roamed the tilting decks without a limp; although obedient for the most part, Bill's excitability was more expansive than the normal range of human experience and, at times, spilled into fits of violence. Occasionally he sat in a trance, prompting the obscure and almost menacing aside that this man 'acts strangely'.

Feeble and brain-addled, Bill arrived back home to Melbourne, a casualty of war before he'd made the Western Front. Back on land, he seemed befuddled. At times he confounded his medical examiners. Had he been to France, they interrogated repeatedly. He couldn't answer. What work might he like to do? He didn't know that either.

Bill's eyes looked down upon his hands; one was scarred. He couldn't recall when or how it was damaged. At every turn Bill was a baffling conundrum. His doctors swayed between a kind of sympathetic understanding of his plight and the harder-edged conclusion that there was a whiff of malingering. Regardless of such professional pontificating, Bill was a changed man: sometimes listless, sometimes roaring at his inquisitors. At times, after a momentary flourish, he'd slump back and sit quietly, wasted, refusing to take in food.

Frustrating his doctors, Bill was cross-examined: if he showed no eagerness to return to his previous work then what might he like to do with the rest of his life? Of that, Bill was certain, and wrote: 'uncertain'.

Bill was dosed up with a concoction of 'triple bromides'— a standard sedative mix of the day—and admitted to hospital.

His doctors tried to slot him into a box: the diagnoses flew about, trying to hit their mark. He was reported as having concussion but no evidence was forwarded. At other times he was reported as being clear of fits; whether these were fits of violence or epilepsy is never clear, but more likely the former. Was it shell shock, the doctors asked. But there was no evidence that he reached France or was near any exploding shells of any kind. Meningitis, perhaps? The evidence was illusory. The medical fraternity scratched about, like chooks in a henhouse, seeking a diagnosis; none was forthcoming.

Sometimes Bill spoke in a distant, dreamy manner, as if his body had returned from overseas but his mind still wandered abroad. He told his doctors that he recollected leaving Melbourne but was 'unable to remember anything on the other side', as if 'the other side' was some ethereal place for lost souls.

Flummoxed, the doctors discharged him home to his parents. But it did not last, and his despondent father, unable to cope with Bill's oddities, trudged back to the hospital with his son in his wake. On arrival at the hospital, an unconcerned Bill blithely gave away all his personal belongings.

In December 1917, three months after he had landed back in Melbourne, Bill was formally discharged from the Australian Army as medically unfit and sent home again.

The Repatriation Department classified Bill as 100 per cent fully disabled, a conclusion one would have thought was not too difficult to arrive at.

Six months later, Bill forlornly wrote: 'I have been unemployed since discharge. My present state of health is as follows: Cerebro-spinal meningitis. I suffer from pains in back and severe headaches. Shell Shock.'

Two weeks after writing this, Bill vanished from his father's care; hot-headed, he grabbed a car and drove several hours from Melbourne to Bendigo, reckless and oblivious to cost. Bill, despite his disjointed mind, had the wits to steal money from a friend in Bendigo. In his turbulent wake came the police. They reported him as 'mentally affected' and 'missing for two weeks . . .'

Bill was arrested as a public nuisance, returned to Melbourne, and taken to Royal Park Receiving House, the major psychiatric reception centre in the state of Victoria. In an obliterating gesture Bill was labelled as 'mental', explaining nothing, yet apparently everything.

Bill bubbled into Royal Park, all affability, and casually confessed to his doctors that he had attacked his brother violently over a trifle, and then took a motor car from Melbourne to Bendigo. He was 'voluble and talkative; inordinately self-satisfied [and] appears to have no sense of the seriousness of his position. His own account of himself exhibits evidence of most erratic conduct and loss of self-control ... And with regard to the civil charge hanging over him he seems to regard himself as the injured person. Ward reports show him to be "simple" and in consequence I have no doubt that he is irresponsible.'

The Inspector-General of the Insane, a title more in keeping with Edwardian militarism than the care of those in such private pain, wrote on behalf of Bill:

> Lunacy Department,
> Melbourne,
>
> 9th August 1918.
>
> 'In re ex-Pte, William Henry Brand, 6618, 7th Battalion,
>
> This lad ... returning to this country as a mental case ... has
> committed a felony in Bendigo.
>   He is allowed out on bail and has to appear at the Supreme
> Court in Bendigo ...
>   There is no doubt that the boy is mentally unstable,
> and in my opinion he should not be held responsible for his
> crime. In the first place it is necessary to rescue him from the
> consequences of his act, and subsequently to put him in some
> position in which he can be prevented from misbehaving in a
> similar manner.
>
> I am,
> Yours faithfully,
>
> W Ernest Jones
> Inspector-General of the Insane

The letter was a slender moment of understanding, and less than one week later, ex-Private W.H. Brand was released from all charges 'as insane'.

Bill was transferred to the nearby Royal Park Hospital for the Insane and confined there for five months. A diagnosis of 'adolescent mania' was made with a nod, probably, to evidence that his illness had roots before adulthood. When he departed the asylum, the Repatriation Department concluded that Bill's incapacity for earning a livelihood was now only three quarters. What this actually meant and how they arrived at this conclusion is never made clear, but apparently with the viable one quarter he had left, Bill was supposed to make a living.

It did not take long for Bill's health to further decay. He wrote— pulling together his splintered mind—and argued for a fairer pension. He complained that in cold weather his gammy leg ached and that he suffered from 'defective vision in the left eye; shooting pain in the region of the heart; giddiness at times'.

Out of hospital he tried the arduous work of horse-breaking as a form of casual employment, giving new meaning to the term 'casual'. But his failing health made breaking horses nigh on impossible.

Living a pinched existence—with no appetite, pain racking his head—at only 25 years of age he presented to the Repatriation Board like an old man: his hands were discoloured blue; his legs leaked pus and his scarred knee was an ever-present reminder of life before the First World War. Sometimes he was giddy and swayed, his memory always fuzzy. England during the war years was more a dream than reality.

To the machinery of government, Bill Brand was an irritant to be extruded. The response was pitiless; his pension was cut.

In appeals for more money, he stated: 'My ground of appeal is that I am suffering from effects of Gas and spine troubles' (although there is no evidence of any 'Gas' exposure during the war). The scar on his right hand, of which previously he could not recall the cause, was now recorded as a gunshot wound. The truth was that Bill was mentally ill. Gusts of mania knocked him about and imagined voices pestered him.

Bill was up against it whenever he applied for reconsideration of his pension—military custom, misplaced medical certitude, and the inertia of indifference conspired against him. Whenever he asked for a raise, it was with the wavering conviction of a man accustomed to rebuke. Each rejection rankled. In many ways his pension battle was the real war that Bill waged, not the one he never fought in Europe. It was with the aggrieved air of the misunderstood—the eternal lot of the mentally ill—that Bill put pen to paper.

In 1923, Bill's life changed unexpectedly when, against all the odds, he met and married a girl with the enchanting name of Pearl Patten. Bill was smitten by Pearl, whose delightfully alliterated name charmed all before her. Pearl was a working-class girl who laboured at the local Pelaco shirt factory and Bill was lucky to find her. Family history has it that Pearl's brother, Gordon—a carpenter like Bill—brought Bill home from work to meet Pearl. It was a match made not so much in heaven as in rough-hewn Richmond, an inner-city suburb of Melbourne. To the Patten family he was always 'Bill'.

Pearl was a nurturing woman—by instinct and necessity; she became the sole carer for her younger brothers after their father abandoned the family, and her mother died young. We can only imagine that Bill was, at best, an unsteady suitor. But in a Richmond terrace, on a summer's day in early 1923, Bill and Pearl married.

When Bill came into Pearl's life, the family oral history is that Pearl latched on to him for security; in that assessment she would be terribly wrong. One year after marriage Bill was driving cars for a living but sometimes worked as a wood machinist or gardener or labourer for extra money, but often there was nothing. He fronted up for another medical assessment and was depressed, thin, coughing and blue; repeatedly tested for tuberculosis and syphilis, nothing was found.

Over the next few years, despite marriage, Bill was a mess.

His right leg, so long an aggravation to him, scarred and swelling, had now atrophied and was smaller in circumference than the left. Chilblains appeared on his ears—minor but painful—telling of his poor lot in life. From within the foul innards of his lungs he coughed up phlegm at will. The tips of his left middle and left index fingers were sliced off in a factory accident.

In 1929, when the world was highly irrational and about to trip into depression, Bill was noted at his annual check to be 'rational and though mildly euphoric has no mental disorder'. On the edge of an apocalyptic world, Bill was considered saner than most. But his wife saw otherwise as their home life fell apart. She implored his doctors to help and wrote to them trying, in vain, to understand her husband's affliction. Her voice, as we read her words, betrays a rising tide of fear; of not knowing what to make of a man so twisted and unreasonable.

By 1931 the doctors recorded that Bill had several false teeth, and was nervy and tremulous; the two puncture marks at the base of his spine from his time in an English hospital were still visible. His left ankle was bloated with infection and he woke from dreams at night awash in sweat.

Bill suspected his wife might leave him. His doctor chimed in: '[Bill] has some emphatic views regarding his wife, probably delusions regarding her fidelity, but he denies this.' Bill was squeezed by the pincer of cold bureaucracy and the threat of a departing wife.

With military understatement, it was recorded that Bill's 'dress and manner is rather unusual' when Bill swanked about in two pairs of women's silk stockings. Bill was not seen as psychiatrically unwell and, almost unbelievably, scornfully, his doctor wrote: 'I cannot state there is any definite disorder in this man. He is a constitutional psychopath, very cunning and plausible.' Bill was a loafer, to his accusatory eyes.

In calling Bill a psychopath, his doctor was really calling Bill a malingerer—suggesting that his apparent mental illness was fake. And with that supernatural gift of the army doctor, Bill's disability was assessed as a mere twelve per cent from his wartime duty. Although feelings of insurrection may have swelled in Bill's breast, he had little choice but to accept.

On a Monday night, while in the Army general hospital, as if to put his twelve per cent assessment to shame, Bill absconded from his ward and waltzed into 'a picture show'. The movie, in 1931, would have begun with the obligatory singing of the imperial anthem 'God Save the King'. In the midst of this throng of seated, orderly movie watchers was William, Bill, Billy, or whatever he called himself that night, disorderly and ready to combust. The national anthem, it seems, was not enough singing for Bill in his manic state, and, clad only in his pyjamas, he stood unabashed and raucously sang to the cinema audience. The syllables spilled from his lungs as he entertained those about him. At moments like these, Bill saw himself as impregnable.

Mania, at its purest, can seem to be a liberating force. It offers a release to pursue what we all spontaneously desire, but curb. When manic, Bill was a froth of rascally notions, and when his mind unzipped, words streamed through the breach as compressed high-energy packages that whizzed about and took aim at everything in his sights. When manic on full throttle, Bill was ablaze. Even in rare moments of apparent solace, beneath the surface bubbled oddity: ladies' silk stockings continued to be his preferred leg attire.

The following years offered no prolonged periods of what anyone would regard as normalcy. Exiled from the normal run of life, he scrapped about for jobs. His relationship with the army was one stumbling inconvenience after another: 'I seem to have misplaced my papers while out fishing'; 'Can you please replace my lost file?'; 'Would you kindly forward a copy of my discharge papers?' In peace, as in war, Bill was a pestering distraction for the army.

Bill's marriage did not last; not a surprising outcome. Indeed it is extraordinary to think it persisted seven years, testimony to the values of the time to marry for life regardless of the suffering incurred. For some time Pearl held tight and maintained a dignified silence. But like so many other spouses married to men returned from the war and with mental illness, Pearl was unable to absorb the extremities of Bill's mood and his threats of violence. Family history has it that on one occasion, she awoke in fright to find the dark silhouette of her husband standing over her, looking at her with a fixed stare. Pearl, bewildered, went to Bill's doctors for help; they offered little. Whatever tender pull of affection she had once felt had long vanished. According to family lore, Bill's father, concerned for the safety of his daughter-in-law, urged Pearl to flee. And so Pearl, taking this advice, bundled together her belongings and self-respect and fled, finding refuge elsewhere. It is hazy as to when she left Bill, but it was probably around 1930; when she did she took their young adopted daughter.

By October 1931 Bill was receiving a pension of 2/2/-, Pearl 13/11 and their adopted daughter 6/-. Bill reported to the Repatriation Board, dutifully, that he did not reside with Pearl or his daughter, but had financially supported both since 'wife deserted him about 12 months ago. Address of wife unknown.'

In 1932, Bill sat down and tried to write a summary of the previous fifteen years of his life. For us, it fills in lost years, much of it grubbing about seeking employment: of his time as a handyman at a hotel in New South Wales after discharge from the army; working at Appelton's Tannery in Richmond for eight months where the fumes—rising from an acid cauldron in which animal hides were pickled—scraped his lungs raw; at Johnson's and Morrison's of Burnley, where his two fingertips were sliced clean off; labouring at Larkin Aircraft Co. for two years until 1927 and of his inevitable sacking when staff were cut; and the many odd jobs he sought and sometimes did, and of countless disagreements with bosses. Bill had neither style nor connections to help leaven the blows.

In the March of 1933 he was boarding in an outer Melbourne suburb, and, unsurprisingly, created trouble. Neighbours, fearful, reported to the police a man doing 'peculiar things'. This time, Bill had set about trying to purchase a car but, of course, he had no money. Bill had left the care of his parents, stating he, 'does not get on with his father who wants to treat him "like a small boy"'. Despite this, the police called for his father—the one constant support in

Bill's life. His careworn father attended but Bill had 'a wild look in his eyes' and stalked about, raving and howling, swinging his arms extravagantly. To the police he seemed shrunken in physical stature, thinned out, and his spindly legs and wild features gave him the appearance of a starved bird of prey. His neighbours, frightened, drew back.

The following year Bill sank from his manic elevation and, ground down, became profoundly depressed. He remained in this depressive torpor for months; his talk slowed, each viscous syllable prised, hard-won, from his mouth.

In 1934 there were no specific treatments for melancholic illness. It was a matter of nursing care, physical exercise, water baths, nourishment, and gently tending to the torments of men and women who saw no hope of resurrection of their spirits. Those severely affected by melancholia sometimes fantasised that their brains were rotting, their bowels unmoveable and that life was a farce in need of obliteration.

When Bill was assessed, a shellshock specialist, Dr Clarence Godfrey, pronounced him as 'very mental', a seemingly more vigorous denunciation than Bill's previous label of just 'mental'. It was noted also that Bill had a peculiarly shaped head and that in his malnourished head only two teeth remained.

When his depression broke, Bill returned to his parents. Unexpectedly, his wife, Pearl, briefly reappeared in early 1934 and wrote to the authorities:

> I desire to appeal on behalf of my husband. He is suffering from
> Neurasthenia and mental trouble. I had to leave him owing to
> his violence some time ago. I returned to him a few months ago,
> but owing to his mental condition I have had to leave him again.

She wrote again, asking that a full pension be granted and mentioning that she had been forced to leave and travel to a small town and find work to support her child and herself: 'I have commenced a home on two occasions and have found it impossible to continue owing to my husband's mental state. I am really afraid that something may happen.'

Her pleas were met with indifference; Bill's pension went unchanged. Pearl cut herself adrift, and seems to have made no further contact with her husband.

And then, an unusual letter landed on the desk at the Repatriation Department towards the end of 1934. It was a query from a woman in country Victoria, 'whether there was any truth in a rumour that . . . [Bill Brand] . . . was dead'. The correspondent stated 'that her son went to the War with Mr Brand, and he had heard that Brand was deceased'. The enquirer further noted that Mrs Brand 'had given it out that her husband had died some months ago, and had remarried'. So a rumour was about that Bill was dead. When you tidy away the mentally ill, the tidiest of all methods is to kill them off. That's what happened to Bill. Although Bill didn't have the wherewithal to counter the claim, the army did. The enquirer was politely told that Bill Brand was alive.

Bill was still capable of the odd gardening job but for the most part his catalogue of illnesses festered. At the end of 1935, Bill's already mutilated left hand was 'bitten by another man' although how and where this occurred remains a mystery; no happy circumstance could have led to this. Bill's afflicted hand was bandaged and he requested admission to hospital; it was denied. When he requested more money, it was denied.

Hospitals might be for the sick but they are also shelters for the lost and lonely and are places of social refuge. Often Bill wanted nothing more than safety, and just a little company.

A depressed mood bit Bill hard again in late 1938. This time Bill became agitated about his mother, a revolving theme whenever he was low, and was convinced that some lurking evil force was about to steal 'her house from her'. The attending doctor struggled to extract answers from Bill's sluggish brain as Bill's thoughts trickled into speech; patient and doctor waited for the melancholia to thaw. Bill sat and stared and every so often mouthed the following sentence: 'One has to be always in the warning for other people.' The doctors had no idea what he was on about; depressed and beset by guilt—so characteristic of such black moods—a delusional Bill uttered that he ate only small portions of food 'so that the poor people may have enough'.

Five months later, in May, Bill's sister Mary was found dead in an outside toilet in a suburban backyard in Fitzroy, a gunshot wound to her head. Mary was often unwell and suicidal. Her employer remembered her as:

> hysterical and she had to be held down . . . She had been in
> Royal Park under observation for mental trouble . . . depressed
> and unable to concentrate . . . Once she put a sheet around her
> neck and pulled it with her hands . . . the other [time] she was
> about to open an upstairs window and she said she was going
> to throw herself out; [she] told [a doctor] that she often felt like
> throwing herself under a tram.

In the early days of the Second World War Bill was back as a munitions worker, constructing weapons of war in Footscray. Even disturbed, his abilities as a machinist were in demand. His weary mother dragged her son to the Army Outpatients for review. She complained that Bill had been 'calling that someone is calling for help. He wanders at night.' Throughout the assessment Bill sat still and said little. Unable to care for himself, he heard the voices of his brothers and other people while with the doctor.

Just after Christmas he collapsed into despair again and confessed that 'he generally breaks down at Christmas on account of memory of previous unfortunate Christmas happenings'. His nutrition was poor, but his early life of horse-breaking and carpentry left him with a stringy muscularity. He was briefly admitted to a medical ward in the Repatriation Hospital, but straight away absconded—absent without leave (AWOL)—a repetition of his first escapade in England in 1917. When he returned, the bone-headed military response was to discharge him.

One of his doctors wrote, in an echo of a previous diagnosis:

> I do not think that this ex-soldier is certifiable. He is a constitutional psychopath ... cunning and not truthful ... [his] statements cannot be accepted as reliable. Should not be admitted to Hospital: treatment useless.

It seems another wrong diagnosis and contemptuous conclusion; the army's blind and cruel manner of dealing with Bill had not altered one jot over 25 years.

Given that his doctors had not twigged to his state of mental illness, Bill offered them a clue, articulating that his head seemed tight, and indeed that he had no head at all. Amazingly, against the grain of common—but not apparently military—sense, his army doctor concluded: 'He is undoubtedly "strange" but ... not certifiable.'

And so it remained that Bill, who had never been *quite right* since he landed in England in 1916, was now, 25 years later, an object of medical curiosity: not quite mad enough to be incarcerated yet not sane enough to live with others.

Bill rummaged about the streets of Melbourne, impecunious and vulnerable, a combination of attributes that made him prey to the unscrupulous. Trouble soon came. In 1941 Bill was arrested in St Kilda and committed to Pentridge Gaol on criminal charges: forging Savings Bank passbooks. His brother pleaded for Bill's release, arguing that his misfit brother was not responsible for his actions. Bill remained in gaol awaiting medical review.

The case was given some prominence and reported in the Melbourne newspaper *The Age*:

Suffered from Shell Shock

Whether his age was 50 or 61 was a matter of doubt to William
Henry Brand, Acland Street, St Kilda, machinist, who came up
for sentence before Judge Clyne ... yesterday. Brand pleaded
guilty last week to having forged and uttered a State Savings
Bank passbook, and a jury found him guilty on two counts of
perjury ... He gave his age yesterday as 50, but Judge Clyne
pointed out that his counsel said his age was 61 ...

The presiding judge, taking into account Bill's parlous psychiatric
state, released him on a three-year good behaviour bond of twenty
pounds and ordered that Bill report to a Major Inglis of the Salvation Army. In handing down his finding, the judge noted the vile
actions of Bill's neighbours, who, it seems, sensing Bill's vulnerable
mental state, exploited him for monetary gain.

Among the pages of Bill's medical and army dossiers are the twigs of
this carpenter's life: the smallest splinters of information that remind
us that he was a man who, illness aside, simply had to get through
each day. On one page is a list of numbers, so unprepossessing and
apparently anonymous that one is tempted to flick over them to get
to something juicier. But the list on this page makes Bill all the more
human. It is a list of all of his unpaid tram fares, carefully documented by the Repatriation Department, and awaiting payment: a
sad vestige of a hard life.

September 1943 found Bill ranting and threatening his parents.
The police, yet again, were called to apprehend him. Dropped off at
the Army General Hospital, Bill, who hadn't slept for 24 hours, was
promptly given a sedating elixir of bromides and phenobarbitone (a
powerful anti-epileptic drug). By 4 am he was still awake. During the
night he did all manner of strange things: slipping his coat on and
off and on again as if in a private game with himself, and prancing
about the ward, swiping at imaginary flies; when placed in his bath,

he swished the water about and played 'trains' in a world of his own making like a small child.

The following day, uncooperative, Bill flipped through ridiculous ideas so rapidly no one could follow him. At night he shot out of bed and danced in the rain. When he was grabbed and manhandled back into the dry, he spat irrational volleys of words at his attendants; among them he stated, rationally, that he was still married, though his wife had long since gone, her loss a scar he never erased.

Bill's doctors certified him as a lunatic, and police dragged him to Bundoora Mental Hospital, where his life was about to undergo a change.

On admission to Bundoora, Bill was a muttering mess, uttering a lingo only comprehensible to him. At times, when questioned, his rank of private and his regimental number were all he could summon from his army life, snatches of memory from a perforated past. He drew his psychiatrist's attention to the twittering birds that perched on the eucalypts outside. Bill, confidentially, revealed that the birds and beasts of the bush conveyed cryptic messages to him. These he understood. And sometimes he confessed, as if he had committed a crime, that among the squawking and growling he could hear the whispers of his dead father calling him.

The haunting image of the asylum lunatic hung heavily in post-war Australia. The most famous of all the Victorian-era psychiatrists—the Englishman Dr Henry Maudsley—famously pronounced: 'When a person is a lunatic, he is a lunatic to his finger nails.' Bill—chattering, filthy, unstoppable—was a lunatic to his eight remaining fingernails. Bill's life was all cut up. At every turn, his life had been buggered by genetics, by love, by medicine, by war. He was (to perfection) what the outside person deeply and secretly feared about becoming insane.

18

Bill Brand was a scoundrel in the asylum. He was notorious among the nurses and attendants, and regarded as the most grubby and pesky of patients. As a result, they gave him his own special name.

Asylum patients were commonly stripped of their Christian names and, instead, staff bellowed out their surnames. Bill Brand was shorn of both Christian name and surname: when summoned for breakfast or lunch or dinner, the attendants called out for 'Monkey', rendering Bill more simian than human.

When he felt the call of mischief, Bill aka 'Monkey', might grab a passing taxi and take off to Melbourne, and swan about racking up fares until he was 'recaptured' by some sweating attendant or tumbled out at the asylum gates by the taxi driver. Or he might divert his rowdy spirits into the manic mowing of a patch of the asylum lawn, striding back and forth over the same strip of dirt, hollering for the world to hear until his hazy outline was lost in a locust swarm of grass clippings.

Everyone knew Bill in the asylum, but whether John Cade knew of Bill's trials with the Department of Repatriation, of his feeble begging for money, of the wife who'd left him, or of his adopted child, we don't know. In 1946, the medical and nursing notes often remained mute on patients' lives beyond the asylum walls. So when Bill came under John's care, it was to Bill's mental state that John cast his mind.

Of Bill, John wrote:

His mental state has remained unchanged over the last two
years. He is chronically euphoric: excitable, restless and has no
power of concentration whatever; so lacking even momentary
attention that questions usually fail to interrupt his flight of
ideas. He is dirty and destructive; noisy both day and night.
A rubbish gatherer and petty pilferer.

Soon after he wrote this, John decided to treat Bill with electroconvulsive therapy—a brutal treatment in 1946.

At the time, this kind of therapy was given raw, without the
present-day modifications that smooth out its violent and gruesome
aspects. But at the time, electroconvulsive therapy was the high-
watermark of effective treatments in psychiatry and used for just
about anything on offer.

The essence of the treatment was to bring about an epileptic fit
in the man or woman suffering from psychiatric illness. John knew
about convulsive therapy from his days at Beechworth. There, such
fits were brought about by injecting a chemical into the patient's
bloodstream and waiting until the brain, irritated and prodded
by such a foreign intrusion, launched into a full-blown epileptic
convulsion. By 1946, the chemical injection had been replaced by
an electrical current to do the same job. How these blasts of electricity helped someone was unclear. But there was no doubt that some
patients underwent spectacular improvement.

Preparing a patient for electroconvulsive therapy ran to a strict
protocol; indeed, everything about asylum care in the post-war period
was rigidly run. And with 'Major' Cade at the helm, the Bundoora
asylum ran to the click of a metronome. It takes little imagination to
picture what took place, as Bill was prepared for this treatment.

On the morning of the first treatment, Bill would not receive
breakfast and, if he was in an agreeable frame of mind, bowels and
bladder were emptied; if not, the procedure would still push on.
The thinning scalp hair over his left and right temple would then be

shaved and cleansed with a swab. That's where the electrodes would sit. The electrodes—two flat metal discs, two inches in diameter—were then strapped to the head, one electrode over the left temple, the other over the right.

These two glistening metal discs would be wired up to an apparatus that sat on a table next to the patient. This was the electrical kit—an assemblage of dangling wires, battery and series of switches—that delivered the current to the patient. At the centrepiece of this jumble was a large circular Bakelite telephone dial, to ring up the length of time the current would flow.

Bill would be asked to lie on his back on the treatment bed, while a quintet of nurses gathered about him, the first four each holding down one of his limbs. With arms and legs pinioned, a fifth attendant would place a gag in Bill's mouth and carry out the task of firmly pressing down on Bill's forehead, keeping the head hard upon the pillow. This was to stop his head bucking forwards when the electrical current was applied; such violent head movements had been known to crack the vertebral column.

At the appointed time, with each attendant gripping their assigned body part, the doctor rotated the telephone dial, twiddled with a knob or two, and a short blast of electricity would surge into Bill's body—rendering him unconscious, a merciful release from any memory of that moment.

The next phase was remarkably choreographed.

Immediately after Bill blacked out, his torso would have buckled and thrust upwards from the bed, head snapped back hard and jaw clenched, his entire body locked in a mass of contracting muscle, like some hideous and twisted slab of stone.

Next, the body would break into shuddering violent movements, limbs rocking back and forth, each threatening to tear itself out of its socket along the seam that held it fast to the torso, but kept in place and subdued by the firm grasp of the attendants at each station. This agitation of flesh and bone continued, perhaps for a minute or two until, drained, the body went limp, the mind stilled and the sweating attendants released their hold.

This was electroconvulsive therapy in 1946. Treatments were given to a patient two or three times a week—sometimes more frequently.

John Cade wrote that Bill 'had nine ECT treatments [with] remarkable improvement. He is now quiet, clean and tidy in his appearance, well behaved and an excellent and willing worker.'

Bill's mental state remained settled over the next few months, despite the occasional oddity, such as his request to wear sunglasses about the asylum grounds. Improved enough, he was sent on leave but trouble soon stirred. While he stayed with his parents, a 'friend rang on behalf of the ex-soldier, stating latter is "going off his head"'. An ambulance, now presumably well acquainted with Bill Brand's address, was summoned and he was taken to the Repatriation General Hospital in Caulfield. Bill breezed back into the wards and—bypassing social etiquette—chatted to his old doctors on a first-name basis. Mentally aloft but physically worn, Bill resumed what he saw as his exalted position and boasted of his accomplishments, though we can't imagine what they might have been. He wandered about the hospital but soon his irrational and disconnected thoughts twisted into persecutory notions and he threatened hospital staff. He was injected with the sedative paraldehyde, an act so familiar to him that he must have known what was about to take place next. His exasperated doctor wrote in piqued finality that 'No treatment is likely to do any good', and with that Bill was bundled into an ambulance and despatched back to Bundoora Mental Hospital.

When Bill's mental state continued to slide, John Cade elected to trial more electroconvulsive therapy. Disappointingly, the shock therapy, which had temporarily improved his state on previous desperate occasions, did not help. A month later Bill slid into a permanent state of disordered, garrulous mania: the dirtiest street urchin in an asylum of urchins. By the end of 1947, Bill had been 'in a state of chronic mania' all year.

The two Cade boys—Jack and David—were ten and eight years old in 1948. They loved Bill and called him Monkey without any self-conscious restraint. They had known Bill for two years and were familiar with his outrageous antics:

> We probably saw more of Monkey than Dad. Monkey did things like squeeze the toothpaste out all over the bathroom mirror and put nasty things between the sheets in people's beds and be delighted when they reacted. Things like that. Nothing malicious.
>
> I think Monkey was the main one who helped set the rabbit traps down near the creek. He also took us fishing to the little creek. The plan was to blow up some fish. There was lots of redfin down there. Nothing ever came of it.

Jack and David met Bill weekly after every Sunday concert: 'We'd file out and meet up at the same spot.' The three of them sat on a bench, a typical park bench, about 50 metres from the Cade house on a slope looking towards the asylum wards. Bill would sit in the middle, Jack and David on either side of him:

> He talked quickly, loudly; lots of jokes and puns. He was happy to be with us; was kind to us; we weren't frightened one bit. He talked, at times, to non-existent people and did so fluently. I'd look around for the recipient of Monkey's talk but there was never anyone.

The two boys devoured Bill's offerings, wide-eyed, knowing instinctively when eccentricity merged into insanity and when to step back. When they sat down they didn't have long to wait for Bill to concoct a story; indeed it was the same story every week.

From a brown paper bag that jutted from the side pocket of his soiled suit coat, Bill pulled out, like a conjuror, his weekly treat for the boys: 'They were always humbugs ... black-and-white striped ones. We'd suck on them like there was no tomorrow.'

The humbugs, candy-coated capsules—like the casing of some enlarged tropical beetle—glistened and sparkled in the sunlight as Monkey plucked them from the bag. The boys received one each. The big, hard-boiled lollies lolled about the boy's mouths, gathering scoops of saliva until their mouths overflowed. Then Bill channelled a directive from God and whispered to them, gravely: 'Boys, they're poisonous, you know.'

And in a hushed tone: 'And if you swallow, you'll die.'

But Monkey, the Supreme Being with a direct pathway to God, had a strategy to help the boys extricate themselves from death's path. He instructed Jack and David that the only solution was not to swallow the sticky goo collecting in their mouths but to lean forward, crane their necks, and allow the venom to trickle from their mouths and spill to the earth. So the two boys, in unison, would bend their necks forward, open their mouths, and allow a pool of spittle to collect at their feet until it could be said a small lake had formed.

'You had to spit out the juice! And we believed him!'

'Nothing was ordinary with Monkey. It was great fun, we loved it and we loved him.'

Monkey's tales enthralled the boys. He brought to them the voyages of his roaming mind and his jangly words excited and refreshed the ordinariness of the world about them. His mania, rich and succulent, illuminated their world.

For the first time, perhaps in decades, Bill Brand was not leashed to a bed, or laughed at, or belted, or spat upon as he had been in a world that cared little and understood his illness not at all. With the Cade boys he was neither beggar nor thief. To the boys he was an incandescent figure shedding light in their world. The boys saw charm, not threat.

For the rest of the week, Bill scuttled around the wards, rodent-like, from dormitory to pantry to the outside, seeking food and goodies wherever he could find them or steal them or barter them. His hands—fluttering appendages—were constantly moving, touching, stroking and beseeching, and pickpocketing what they might.

By the start of 1948, Bill Brand had been in a state of mania for close to five years. Never a powerful man, he bore little meat on his bones. When his fizzing maniacal energies were spent, he sat, depleted; sometimes huddling in a corner, eyes sunken and thoughts distant, the soft breath of life just visible.

The remnant of a near-demolished human being, Bill was a wreck by the time John Cade resorted to giving him lithium.

When John made the decision, there was no hand of convention to thwart him, nor was there a whiff of an ethics committee to question his action. Nothing could stall John except his conscience. And this, he felt he had answered.

The first evidence we have that John might select Bill as his first subject comes in a brief chemical annotation written on 6 March 1948. He noted that Bill's blood uric acid was 'extremely high'. John believed, from his guinea pig experiments, that he had found evidence implicating uric acid in the state of mania, evidence we now know was false. And in his mind, he felt that administering lithium to Bill might induce the state of tranquillity he had observed in his guinea pigs.

Just over two weeks later, John took the step that was the culmination of work that had first stirred in his mind on the voyage home from Changi three years earlier.

Gathering all the strands of Bill's case, he condensed them and, like a military leader, made a final push into alien lands:

Bill Brand, age 51, chronic mania of about five years' duration. Fair but temporary improvement after ECT two years ago. Since November '46 has completely reverted to his usual state— noisy, restless, untidy and mischievous.

One afternoon in the second half of March, John returned home after his routine ward rounds. It had been an intense day at Bundoora and he was flustered and preoccupied. His wife recalled

that there was 'trouble in the hospital' and patients were 'stirring up'
on the wards. Cade returned to his shed and made up a solution of
lithium citrate.

It is unlikely that John bothered to discuss lithium with Bill's
family and we certainly have no idea what, if anything, he said to
Bill before offering the elixir.

We don't know if Bill gulped or sipped the proffered potion, if
he swallowed obediently, or was enticed, even held down. But what
is almost certain is that he had little idea of what he was consuming.
Patient and doctor were as wise or as ignorant as one another as to
what might unfold over the next few weeks.

After administering the lithium, at day's end John walked the
short distance home. It is likely that his routine that evening was
no different to any other day at Bundoora. Indeed John's routine at
Bundoora was so fixed that his children recall it with some precision
60 years later, as did his wife:

> John would come in and the first thing he did was put down his
> bag and go to the pantry and pour out a very large sherry; and
> as he came out of the pantry he had a glass about twice the size
> he should have . . . He had a sip so he wouldn't spill any.

Before dinner he said grace with the family and then, after dinner,
adjourned to the lounge room to sit in the regal oak chair he was
given for his 21st birthday:

David remembers this clearly:

> He sat in this chair every night of his married life; he was a man
> of rituals. He'd sit in that chair sometimes until 2 or 3 in the
> morning if he was reading . . . and much to Mum's chagrin he'd
> still be there in his suit from work.

John's understanding of mental illness was underwritten by his
acceptance of its physical basis. Mania, he thought, might be caused
by an excess of some unknown chemical percolating through the

body; depression caused by a deficit. John had dispensed with Freud, his bête noire, years ago. To John, Freudian fantasies could no more explain manic depression than they could measles. The answer, he was convinced, lay not in our dreams but in our body's chemistry. Giving lithium to Bill was the pragmatic endpoint of all his thinking.

John sat down to record his experiment with lithium on a set of lined cards. The cards, today, are archived in the Medical History Museum at the University of Melbourne, and the detailed notation laid out for us gives us a fascinating glimpse into John Cade's mind. A man of few idle words, he crafted each line. The experiment was probably recorded in his favourite Swan fountain pen, used in Changi.

The man who taught himself how to cut his sons' hair, and how to re-sole his own shoes, wrote on these cards with the precision of snipping bonsai: crisply and pedantically. Post-Changi, nothing was to be wasted in John's world: not paper, not ink, not words. The thin stream of ink from his fountain pen shaped words to reflect his distilled thoughts: each word laid out precisely, mindful of the impact on an observer.

He started writing the first of his cards soon after he gave Bill his first treatment:

29/3/48: Commenced lithium citrate mixture 10 grains thrice a day. After a few days increased to 20 grains thrice a day and then for a few days to 40 grains thrice a day—commenced to vomit and complain of nocturnal enuresis [bed-wetting]. Mental state improving. Dosage reduced and still sensitive so discontinued and replaced with capsules of lithium carbonate 5 grains twice a day [one grain is the equivalent of 64.8 mg].

His notes point to an early improvement in Bill. One might have anticipated eagerness to express satisfaction, or something akin to excitement in these lines. But no. John's emotions, severely clipped by three and a half years in Japanese hands, remained buttoned down.

As early as the fourth day of treatment, John wondered if Bill was a little quieter. Jean remembered this moment:

> The attendants were very faithful to John. John had said about his lithium work: 'Now I don't want you talking about this to anyone. If you think so and so is better on the lithium don't say it until we really prove it.' And he used to say to me: 'They're very faithful they're sure Billy's a bit better today but I said don't guess, make sure.'

John recorded that Bill was transferred to Ward 'A', where patients were less disturbed, less disruptive, and reflected that Bill 'had been ill so long and confined to a "chronic ward", [that] he found normal surroundings and liberty of movement strange at first'.

5/5/48:   Has been in 'A' ward for about 10 days and after steadily settling down, now has appeared perfectly normal both to my observation and that of his relatives for over a week. Continues on lithium carbonate 5 grains twice a day.

20/5/48: Continues well.

29/5/48: A little unsettled today. Discontented that he has not been able to go home (housing difficulty). Lithium carbonate increased to 10 grains thrice a day.

30/5/48: Settled down again.

3/6/48:   Lithium carbonate reduced to 5 grains thrice a day.

7/6/48:   Well.

9/6/48:   Lithium carbonate increased to 10 grains thrice a day.

14/6/48: Very well. More self-confidence.

The initial nursing observations had been astute. Each day when John walked into the ward and saw with his own eyes Bill's restored mind and behaviour, doubt vanished, and in that moment of percussive discovery John Cade knew that he had stumbled upon something quite remarkable.

Bill's metamorphosis was as unpredicted as it was exhilarating.

By the last week of June, Bill Brand, as sane as any man on earth, was allowed brief temporary leave from the asylum. Every eddying hallucination that wreathed through his mind, each bizarre thought, and all the grotesque phantasms that had over three decades tormented him, all just simply dissolved into the air. It was as though something mystical had happened and indeed, in times past, Bill might have been revered—or burned—such was the change in his manner. Irritability yielded to beguiling charm, mischief to merriment. The world was about to see a new man transformed by an element of nature, and observe what the young Cade boys, Jack and David, had always intuitively understood about Bill.

John's wife affectionately remembered this time:

> Everyone was very fond of Monkey; yes, it was remarkable. But what amazed me was that his parents and all turned up and dressed him up. I never knew that Bill had any relatives. Visitors just didn't come.

But Bill did have relatives and on this day the consoling hand of his family took their son, their brother, home. With the optimism of life newborn, he greeted his mother and brothers. The Cade boys remember them arriving in a Buick.

It was arranged for Bill to be discharged on indefinite trial leave from the asylum on 9 July 1948.

On that July day, a single penny would buy Bill a small bag of humbugs on the streets of Melbourne; the Australian Immigration Minister, Arthur Calwell, proclaimed that Australia might accept 200,000 Baltic migrants; Melbourne employers bemoaned that modern boys were 'dead-end kids' who 'were poor workers, always looking for the easy way out'; terrorists slaughtered 27 people in Malaysia; and the South Melbourne Swans football team made final preparations for their weekend match.

While the city was busy in myriad ways, Bill, with a stiff breeze at his back, unfurled his spinnaker and set sail from the asylum harbour, relieved of his burden of 30 years. Lithium, a salt of the earth, had found its way into the mind of a man who had lost his. And in so doing, after five years of continuous insanity, Bill Brand stepped out through the asylum gates and into the Melbourne of 1948.

19

Bill was the first to receive this magical elixir, lithium, but he was not the last. Within weeks of starting Bill on lithium, John Cade scanned the asylum grounds and looked for another patient. And then another. His lithium net spread wide.

In this one tiny corner of all the mental hospitals around the world, something incredible was germinating. New growth and hope were nurtured in the most unlikely of places and people. Men, lost to themselves and others in a haze of delusions and hallucinations, returned to a life long forgotten. A transformation in how mental illness was treated was underway.

John's second patient was a man—shorn of his surname—known around Bundoora as P.J. Manic, wild and mutinous, P.J. was in a locked ward. Within a couple of months of starting lithium, P.J. made a miraculous recovery. He started making daily trips into the city of Melbourne like any respectable suburban commuter, and, in an astonishing turnabout, seven months after his first dose of lithium, he was working, steadily, reliably, at General Motors Holden.

A third patient—whose durable mania had burned ferociously for five continuous years—was stripped free of all hallucinations and delusions within nine days of starting treatment. Six months later—now a model employee—he found work in the sub-editor's office at one of the largest newspapers in Melbourne and was pulling in over six pounds a week.

And then there was the spectacular Polish doctor who (you might remember) startled his psychiatrist on hospital admission with handstands and dazzling somersaults, boasting of his unquenchable need for sex. Six days later, on this wondrous stuff called lithium, he was back to his professional self.

Other men—some who'd been padlocked and bolted in single rooms in the hospital, some just garrulous pests—were treated with lithium. These were the vagrants, the tradesmen, and the professional men of Melbourne: all afflicted by the same illness, all captives in the same manic bag. Many of these men had been in and out of asylums their entire lives; all improved to some degree on this fabulous lithium solution, and gave satisfaction to John Cade.

While this blossoming change was taking root in John's hospital patients, Bill Brand remained at home and at work, healthy.

We are never told what work Bill returned to: whether it was the whirring of a lathe at the munitions factory, or the hauling of pickled hides out of an acid broth at the tannery or the clawing at hardened earth with a hoe in a local market garden. Whatever it was, Bill's labour would have been unremittingly hard.

John requested that Bill report back to the Bundoora Asylum in a fortnight's time; and while Bill had never been an exemplary soldier, certainly one that rarely snapped to order on command, he dutifully returned to see Dr Cade in two weeks and continued to do so over the next few months.

The Cade boys remember this buoyant time well, and they kept in touch with 'Monkey'. Or, more correctly, Bill kept in touch with them. For when Bill came into the asylum to be reviewed by Dr Cade, he called in upon the boys. And they set about playing their old game. The three of them sat upon the same wooden bench they'd always sat on; the boys waiting, expectantly, for 'Monkey' to use his magic and pluck a bag of humbugs from his coat pocket so they could play out their well-rehearsed fantasy once again. David still remembers their disappointment:

Monkey seemed to suddenly become less fun when he was better. He had always been a livewire, making jokes, talking quickly and loudly, and to us as kids that was great fun . . . When he came back on one occasion he didn't have any humbugs and he told us that the humbugs were not poisonous.

When the boys, curious and surprised, asked why the humbugs were not poisonous anymore, 'Monkey' spat back with a spark of mischief that lit his eyes: 'That's why they're called humbugs!' But this was only a momentary flash of Monkey's once eccentric wit. Mostly, the flourishing feats of wordplay that had so captivated the boys in past years were gone.

To the rest of the world, Bill Brand had never seemed better, but to the boys there was something sad in this change in their old friend, a loss.

The first sign that something was seriously wrong with Bill came to John in the form of a letter. Bill's family wrote that he had been 'excitable and argumentative' after a 'trivial row'. John wrote back and asked to see Bill. For us, this method of exchange between family and doctor seems excruciatingly slow. But in 1949, a time of starchy formality and unhurried pace, this was the way in which many families contacted the mental hospital doctor.

Bill returned to see John and confessed to ceasing his lithium; John restarted it. Bill returned to his family, but no one was sure if he took his lithium or merely pretended to do so: Bill's truthfulness in the matter was questionable. And then just before Christmas, Bill, having returned home, abandoned (unbeknown to John) his lithium altogether. Mania descended upon him rapidly and on 30 January 1949, his wilting family hauled a sick but spasmodically excitable Bill back to John.

Years later, John recalled this moment when his first lithium patient, Bill Brand, bowled back into Bundoora, as eye-poppingly manic as ever: 'It was the most bitter disappointment of my life.'

John, crestfallen, interrogated Bill. Having assumed he was taking his lithium as prescribed, it was only upon questioning his patient and Bill's brother that John twigged to the truth of the matter: 'I . . . found my former patient had become blasé and had stopped taking his lithium tablets.'

Bill had cherished his leave from the hospital and the liberation from a manic state. But at times he felt physically sick on lithium—a deep pain gnawed away in his abdomen, and the oppression of taking a pill to restore his sanity was a constriction he felt keenly. Lithium had restored Bill's sanity, but when back to normal an incorrigible Bill lost sight of the need to continue taking his medicine.

John decided to re-admit Bill to the asylum. Under close supervision, Bill restarted his lithium treatment. Over the next few weeks the metallic salt seeped back into the ex-digger's body and brain, until three weeks later John pronounced Bill back to 'normal'. As if to display his worth around the hospital, Bill, like a favoured schoolboy, ran errands between wards and did odd jobs for the nursing staff. Bundoora asylum, more than ever, was now his home again.

There were still occasional brief moments when Bill's mind ran off the rails, but by April there was no hint of any mental illness and he remained well for the next six months, pottering about the hospital grounds.

John worked alone on his lithium experiments during the years from 1946 to 1949. No research assistant or medical colleague shared his shed and he certainly invited no one to help him.

Despite this isolation, on several occasions, word got out that he was working with lithium. We know that as early as 1948 John mentioned his fledgling work to fellow psychiatrists at medical meetings. What he said is unrecorded and, like so much of what he did in those years, we are left to speculate. All that is known for sure is that John Cade wanted to work without interference. But his manner and insistence on isolation set up a medical response that was both curious and suspicious as to his activities. It was not long before psychiatrists and administrators dropped in to Bundoora to find out what the elusive Dr Cade was up to, their visits severely irritating him.

Jean remembers the occasional visits from psychiatrists to Bundoora, nosing their way into the Cade household:

> Dr Stoller was the representative of the Army ... he used to come to visit ... and John used to come home and say 'Ah, that Stoller is pretty sneaky ... he's sniffing around, he knows there's something on ... he said the attendance book gives me away. He'd ask: 'What are you on to, John? What are you doing John?' And John said: 'I'll let you know when I know.'
>
> Occasionally people had an idea he might be on to something and they'd use all sorts of methods of asking him: 'I gather you're doing so and so ... do you want any help?'

By the start of 1949, John knew that he had uncovered something remarkable in lithium, and with his once-ill patients blooming with health, he was ready to break this silence and write up his work for publication.

In his research paper, John would argue that lithium, a simple element, could wrangle and tame a specific mental illness—mania. The notion itself was almost unbelievable to many at the time—that lithium, a metal dug from the earth's crust and made into a solution or a tablet, could do this. Even the idea that something inanimate, a godless chemical, could shape a man's mind and govern his behaviour was repellent, even against the natural order, to some doctors. This was a time when the causation of mental illness was in the balance: was it mainly psychological, or biochemical, or perhaps the result of social factors like homelessness and poverty? Many of John's colleagues saw the source of manic depression as stemming from a disturbed family upbringing. To such psychiatrists, it was a mother's malevolent word or a father's brutal fist that twisted a child's upbringing and caused madness. In one motion John was about to challenge these entrenched and cherished beliefs.

John knew that his research article would provoke bitter opposition, particularly among those who were enamoured with Sigmund Freud and psychoanalysis. John had studied but rejected psychoanalysis. John was a practical man who slung a Winchester rifle across his shoulder and who scissored his own sons' hair and who worked in a mental hospital. Psychoanalysis might be fine for the top end of Collins Street, but not in the furnace of an asylum. It had produced negligible success in treating the most severe kinds of mental illness, such as that afflicting Bill. Psychoanalysis would never do for John.

John Cade had long been irritated by Freud and psychoanalysis. Even before the war, the jargon-filled abstractions of psychoanalysis offended him, and over the subsequent years he had sought to cleanse himself of its seductive ideas. To fully understand his criticism, we have to appreciate that John had read Freud extensively. He jotted notes in the margins of the Freudian books he consumed: thoughtful, sharp annotations. John's distaste for Freudian theories is evident in these jottings. On one occasion, he scribbled emphatically: 'Not true. Simply not true.'

By the time he wrote up his lithium experiment on Bill Brand and his other experimental subjects, John had purged himself of Freud and was clear in his thoughts about chemical causation.

John had a set routine for writing up his work. Each night, after dinner, he sat down in his favourite oak chair. The chair was a heavy lump of a thing with two broad flat arms. On top of both arms was a circular hollow (with a carved flower design), just large enough for his mug of coffee. With plenty of room for his nightly glass of sherry, and space for an ashtray next to his coffee mug, John puffed away on his Ardath cigarettes, silently composing his manuscript, ringed by the small pleasures in his life.

The article was to be short and to the point. He thought out clearly what he wanted to say, wiping it clean of anything unnecessary, and, only then, wrote with his Swan fountain pen quickly and with few corrections, until a draft was completed. He had some unusual quirks when it came to writing, and was more than a bit pernickety about the process. John had an aversion to noise, perhaps a troubling residue of the war, but whatever the cause, the Cade household was well-regulated, very neat and never, ever loud. According to Jean, before he sat down to write, John removed any clocks from the room: 'He was funny about clocks, he couldn't study in his armchair with a clock going tick, tick, tick on the mantelpiece. So he'd get up and put [it] in the kitchen.' Even the children's pet fish, swishing around in a glass bowl of water, annoyed him. Out the bowl went too. Once the dining room was silent—banished of all irritants—he could sit meditatively, and compose on paper the events of a momentous year.

Once written, he polished his draft in a manner as unusual as the lithium experiments themselves. In a rather formal way he stood in the dining room, his back towards a corner of the room, and—like a minister of religion in an invisible pulpit—he read his manuscript out loud to Jean, a silent congregation of one. In this manner John Cade preached his paper into perfection.

Cade's historic paper was published in *The Medical Journal of Australia* on 3 September 1949. The paper is a masterpiece, his magnum opus. It is everything a scientific paper should be, and so different to just about every modern scientific paper you will ever read. It is a four-page wonder, a manifesto on the treatment of mania; its scope—of life and death—is operatic. It was published without fanfare—just another article in the midst of hundreds—but it would, in due course, be celebrated as the journal's most cited paper, and for changing the way we think about mental illness.

If you can read English, then you can understand the allure of Cade's paper, and that's the beauty of the thing: anyone can take it in and feel the excitement of the message. It doesn't fall over itself trying to impress; there are no incomprehensible statistics, just simple numbers any primary-school student would understand.

Cade records the lithium treatment of ten manic patients: each one a story. Not all patients treated were a complete success but there are memorable narrative lines of hope in his paper.

By the following month, word was out that a new treatment—concocted in a shed in an asylum in Melbourne—was being used for mania. Collins Street, that haven of private psychiatrists, an address John turned his back on over ten years earlier, came knocking on his door, keen to share their experiences:

> Dear John,
> I have given lithium citrate to two patients with varying
> results. The first patient was a recurrent mania who seemed
> to be remitting when the lithium citrate was commenced.
> Her subsequent improvement was rapid . . .

The second patient was not manic and the effect was less impressive.

Hundreds of kilometres away, in the city of Sydney, the superintendent at Parramatta Mental Hospital, a vast sprawling asylum on the western edges of that city, scribbled a rushed letter to John—a letter of praise, hope and frustration:

> Dear Dr Cade,
> I have been following your work on cases of mania in
> *The Medical Journal of Australia*, and note with interest
> the reference to the use of lithium salts. The drug houses in
> Sydney . . . have been unable to take an order and I should
> be glad if you would advise me of a firm from which they are
> obtainable as I am anxious to use these preparations here.
> Your results, I feel, promise well and may fill one of the many
> gaps in present day psychiatric treatment by relieving a very
> troublesome disorder.
>
> Yours faithfully,
> Dr F.J. Scanlan

Curiosity about John's work was thick in the air. His fellow psychiatrists, who had previously dropped into the Cade home in a desultory manner, now circled *en masse*. John soon felt the prickle of envy. His wife remembered: 'John would say to me, "another sticky beak wanting to know what I'm doing . . . they all seem to have an idea that they can help".'

It seemed to Jean that there was no end of fellow doctors wanting to share the credit for her husband's work. Every status-craving psychiatrist sniffed at John's door to find out what he'd been up to and, like scavenging birds, they flocked about waiting for an opening to snatch their unearned lot.

John, however, was a man shaped by sturdy values sharpened by war; he was never susceptible to the false charms of those circling around him.

Bill Brand remained John Cade's flagship patient, a talisman of lithium's worth. Bill's care and the trajectory of his recovery became a barometer for John and he recorded his clinical progress with more care and detail than any of his other patients.

For the rest of 1949, Bill's home was the Bundoora asylum. At times he experienced a burning abdominal pain and nausea, and occasionally his mind unfurled into mania, and at these latter points he relapsed into a filthy state, foraging about the asylum bins for food. But for the most part, he was well and by the end of September he'd been free of all signs of mental illness for six months.

Bill's entire life had been wayward. Nothing remained smooth for too long before his world capsized, and so it would be on lithium. As he'd done many times before, Bill was about to unravel into loose strings, and dismantle John's hour of triumph. The first indication that Bill was not well came in October, when he was all over the place—sometimes vomiting, his temper testy, and arguing with John about taking his lithium.

John's insistence on prescribing lithium and Bill's resistance to taking it marked their relationship for months. Finally, an uneasy truce settled between the two men—doctor and patient—and John bent to Bill's desires and stopped giving lithium to his patient.

John knew that without lithium Bill would spin off into mania; with it he would remain less manic, but would be physically distressed.

Each successive day while Bill was off lithium, his mental affliction grew. Mania first showed itself in how Bill spoke: each word was a driving rhythmical expression of his rising manic pulse. A single word soon distended into a sentence; a sentence then exploded into a rambling paragraph. Before long, Bill's ungovernable surges shoved his unruly mind into full throttle mania and his sentences flew out, incontinent, without beginning or end.

Within two weeks of stopping lithium, John wrote—taking no joy in the correctness of his clinical prediction of relapse—that Bill was 'At his best manic manner', and back to his old quarrelsome self. John found this relapse and defeat intolerable, and responded by restarting lithium.

John kept escalating the dose of lithium to manage Bill's symptoms. By late November, Bill was taking 40 grains thrice a day—what we now know, nearly 70 years later, is a massive dose of lithium.

But as the lithium dose rose, and John frantically looked for improvement, Bill seemed not to improve a jot. John lamented: 'As noisy and mischievous as ever. It is probable that he is either not taking or quietly rejecting his mixture.' A thin edge of reproach at Bill's likely lack of cooperation can be sensed in John's voice.

Although John continued to pen his descriptions neatly and concisely, there is an air of dismay evident to a reader of his notes over 60 years later. It is the closest we get to seeing John lose control of his meticulously pared-back emotions.

At this point John Cade and Bill Brand both seem exhausted, and a bit fed up with one another. In this slumped state John comments that Bill is now 'saturated at last'. What he meant was that lithium—at its maximum dose—filled Bill's body, soaking every cell and bathing Bill's brain. There was nothing more to give.

But there was a cost to this high dose.

Bill's hands shuddered when he raised a cup to his lips and he wobbled as he walked—both side effects of his lithium treatment. He protested at the taking in of food and lost what little flesh he had on his bones; despondent and weeping at times, only occasionally did he brighten up when John chatted to him. In response to the scrap of a man before him, John reluctantly reduced the lithium dose.

There is a sense of incredible frustration in John's thinking and actions. That having achieved so much with his first patient, he refuses to let go; he won't lose a success that was recently his, and now might just be drifting away from his outstretched grasp.

Two days later John found Bill curled up in bed. His rectum extruded from his body; the pinkish foul protrusion was pushed back in. Sometimes Bill seemed quite well to John. Often he was not.

By the middle of December, against expectations, John reported that Bill was much improved. Rejuvenated, Bill roamed the asylum grounds, and plans were made to give him leave in Melbourne.

Bill had alienated his family with his antics over 30 years, and it was unlikely he could return to them for leave. The problem then, as always, was that outside the asylum there was little warmth and support for the mentally ill. Bill's brutal decades wandering about Melbourne, often lost and sometimes psychotic, were evidence enough of that.

In an effort to change this, a new place of refuge for the mentally ill, a hostel, was opened in Melbourne. *The Argus*, the city's soi-disant leading newspaper, spread the word. No less than the Governor of Victoria, Sir Dallas Brooks, was called upon to open this mental health refuge—named Trelowarren—a slender link between asylum and community. The announcement graced the social pages of the newspaper, wedged above a paragraph announcing that a certain Miss Lillian Guest was to marry a certain Mr Mervyn David (after a 'kitchen tea' of cherry and cream) and below a tribute to Mrs Ivy Wedgwood, Victoria's first woman senator.

Bill took full advantage of this new 'society column' refuge, though its social flutterings in the press were unlikely to have concerned him, and he was transferred there temporarily on 20 January 1950. He returned to his ward at Bundoora after two weeks, apparently bolstered by the experience of Melbourne city life.

As Bill was still quite well in late February 1950, John Cade reduced his lithium to try to reduce the continuing side effects.

In the first week of March, Bill was manic again, his thoughts frothing about. He cursed John and he cursed the medication.

As if scribbling for an unseen jury, which would in future cast a judgemental eye, John Cade wrote, sadly philosophical: 'Under all the circumstances it seems that [Bill] would be better off as a carefree restless case of mania rather than the dyspeptic, frail, little man he looks on adequate lithium.' John, for posterity, then under-lines in his notes: 'Lithium discontinued.'

Bill's manic embers once more ignited.

And again John vacillated. It seems that thoughts flooded in and lathered at the edges of his uncertain mind and again he debated with himself about using lithium. Threading his way through conflicting emotions, he summed up his dilemma: 'His state seems as much a menace to life as any possible toxic effects of lithium.' And so, into the furnace, John casts lithium for the last time, prescribing it on 12 May.

It made little difference. Bill ate almost nothing, and his flesh fell away. His friable skin started to crack and break away like flakes of rust. In his half-demented state, he picked at his skin; infected sores sprang up in crops over his body. His bony wrists and ankles— mere spindles poking out from beneath his sheet—were wrapped in bandages. Odd mannerisms returned: Bill repeatedly ripped off his clothes only to put them on again.

Bill sank into a still state; lithium was stopped. Deep into that night he wafted into lost consciousness. Two partial fits presaged his whole body breaking into a prolonged epileptic convulsion. John, present at Bill's bedside, drew up a syringe filled with phenobarb-itone, and injected the contents into whatever meaty spot he could find in Bill's body. The convulsions stilled. In a final attempt to resurrect Bill, a feeding tube was inserted through one of his nostrils and threaded down his gullet and into his stomach. Badly needed nutrition—probably milk, eggs and broth—was poured in.

Bill was paralysed between life and death, until late in the evening on 23 May 1950 when all trace of life leached away.

Bill lay on his sepulchral bed, the skin of his face—like parchment—drawn over the hollows of his cheeks. He had always had the dimensions of a jockey, but never more so than now, and his miserly 5 feet 5 inches shrivelled into a ball.

To the pathologist who performed the autopsy, Bill was an 'elderly man'. But Bill (to anyone who'd known him) had been 'old' for years. With laughable irony, the pathologist announced Bill's brain as normal, at least normal to the crude means of examining a brain at a pathologist's disposal in the middle of the twentieth century.

The coronial inquest into the death of Bill Brand was held on Thursday 26 October, a cool and cloudy Melbourne day. No one seemed to know Bill's exact age. To the various witnesses he was 50, or 52 or even 54. It was an imprecise way to die.

———

There remained a final twist in Bill's life.

In the month before he died, the Repatriation Board met to consider Bill's application for a full war pension. It was the umpteenth time—over the last 30 years—they'd met to decide on this. In an ironic postscript, the judicial eye of the Repatriation Board accepted Bill as totally and permanently incapacitated from his war service: Bill Brand's pension would be raised to its maximum value. Bill had spent 30 years of his life begging for this pension, but, for Bill Brand, the Repatriation Board's decision was all too late. Official approval came on 25 May, two days after Bill's death, for a payment he would never receive.

At Kennett River, c. 1950. John Cade with David (back), Peter and Jack (front right). (Image courtesy of Cade family)

PART 4

After *the* Face, *the* Hands Reveal Most

FUNNY FARM

Nut farm at most,
To those with money
A Health Resort,
To those who are poor
Medicare Hotel,
For those in the know.
All you need to realise
in Truth and Fact is
it's time out from
Reality,
Sent by the
'Quack'.
Just get better everyone
'Quack, quack, quack'.

*Written by 'J.R.' while in a manic state,
'in tribute to my Doc and nurses'*

...he question of scrap iron for Japan, right any ho...

...was going to be done with it.

...that this Indonesian bid for independence is only... ...head dissatisfaction by the peoples of the East wi... ...ver lordship. The same problem is demanding solu... ...Burma and Indo China... ...of political speculation. Regarding leave, dea... ...at 28 days immediately following disembar... ...k or so in a convalescent camp (probably at Bali... ...over-haul, followed by another 30 days leave... ...are not sure of yet is whether we will get i... ...cumulated recreation leave, which would amo... ...70-80 days. I suppose the department will... ...me as soon as possible - well, they will have... ...and I, darling, are entitled to a pretty good... ...that, I feel so rusty, medically, that I simp... ...if possible three months post-graduate stud... ...like to do a month at St Vincents, a month at t... ...a fortnight at the Eye and Ear, leaving ano... ...swinging - all provided we can keep the depart... ...her to work - as you guessed in one of your ea... ...old brain box is simmering with ideas. I be... ...riod of waiting has allowed many of my no... ...try to crystallise, and I'm just bursting to p... ...test. If they work out, they would represent a g... ...the knowledge of manic-depressive in...

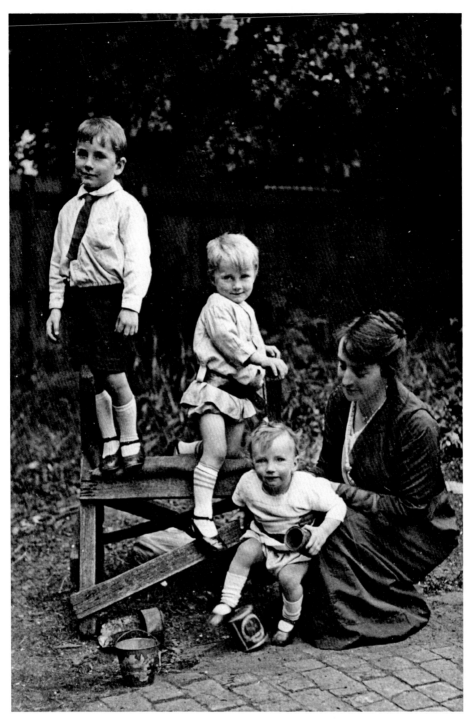

John Cade (left) with brothers David (centre) and Frank, and mother
Ellen, c. 1916. (Image courtesy of Cade family)

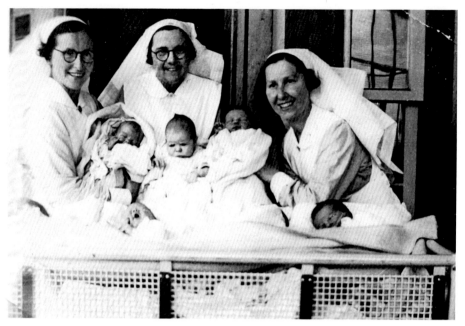

Jean Charles (right) during midwifery training, probably at Women's Hospital, Melbourne, mid-1930s. (Image courtesy of Cade family)

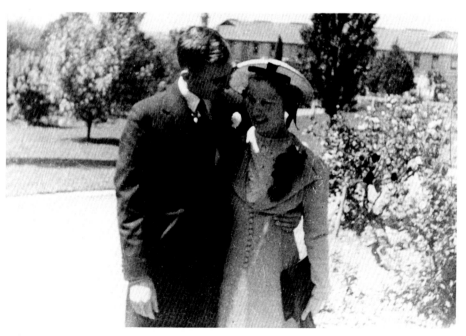

John and Jean Cade in front of Mont Park Mental Hospital on their wedding day, 1 November 1937. Their reception was held in the hospital. (Image courtesy of Cade family)

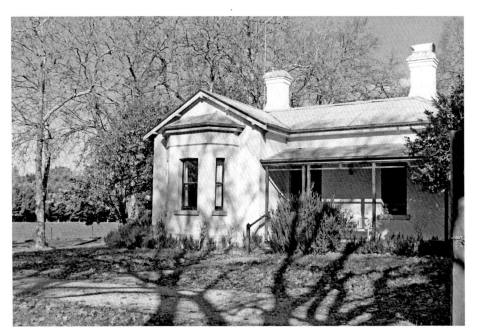

The medical officer's house, Beechworth Mental Hospital, where
John Cade lived as a young doctor early in his psychiatric career.
(Image courtesy of Greg de Moore)

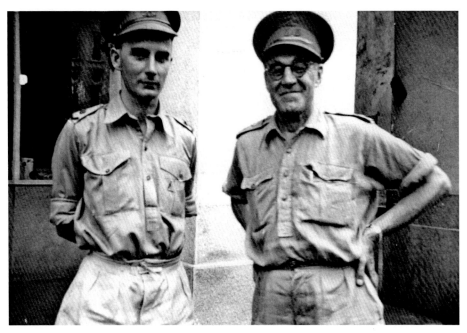

John Cade (left) and fellow soldier R.M.W. Webster, Malaya, 1941.
(Image courtesy of Cade family)

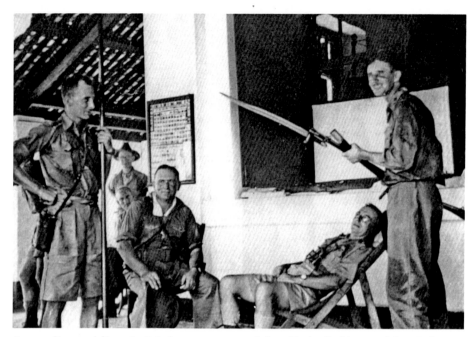

Australian soldiers in Malaya, c. 1941. John Cade (left) watching John Park, who is brandishing a bayonet (right). (Image courtesy of Owen Jenkin)

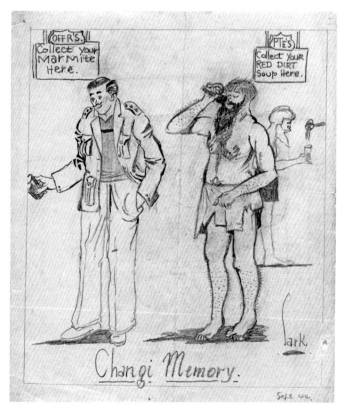

'Changi Memory', drawn by Australian POW Walter Andrew Sarkies, dated September 1944. John Cade was involved in the development of nutritional supplements for the prisoners held in Changi. (W.A. Sarkies collection, State Library of Victoria)

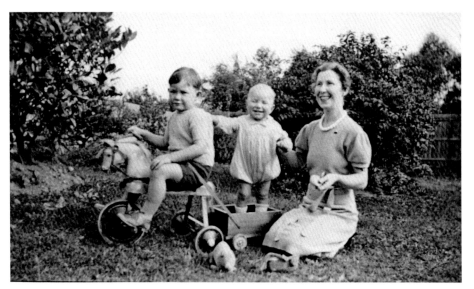

Jack (left) and David with their mother Jean, probably in the back garden of their wartime home in Eaglemont, Melbourne, 1942.
(Image courtesy of Cade family)

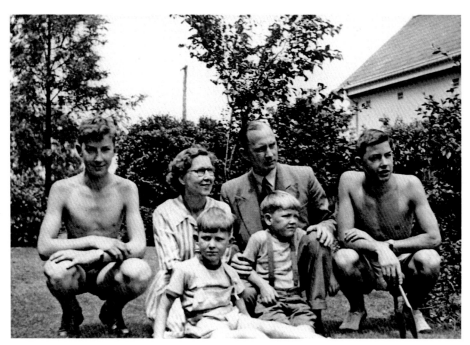

The Cade family in the mid-1950s. Back (left to right): David, Jean, John and Jack. Front (left to right): Peter and Richard. (Image courtesy of Cade family)

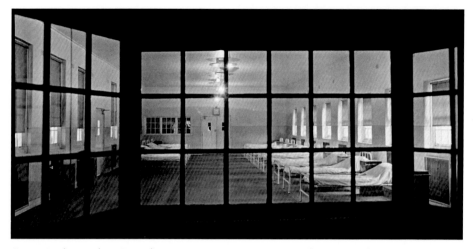

A typical ward in Bundoora Repatriation Mental Hospital, c. 1940s.
(National Archives of Australia)

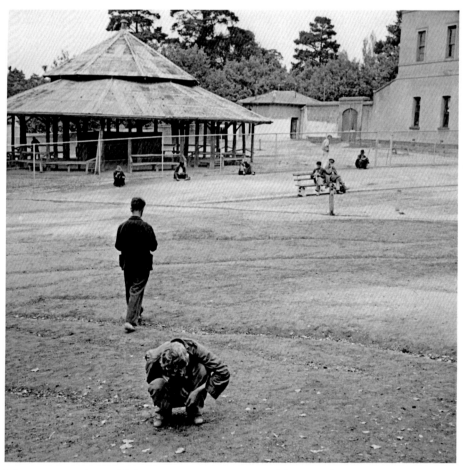

The grim reality of life in a Victorian mental hospital in the early 1950s.
(State of Victoria)

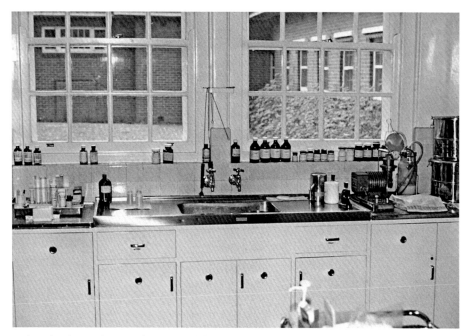

'The shed'—John Cade started his experiments with lithium in the kitchen of an unused ward at Bundoora Repatriation Mental Hospital in the late 1940s. (Image courtesy of Jack Cade)

John Cade began to treat Bill Brand with lithium in 1948. This card records his first few observations. (Image courtesy of University of Melbourne Medical History Museum)

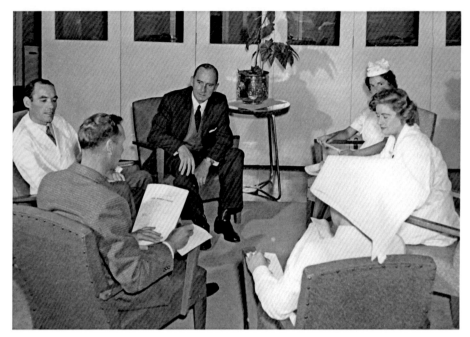

John Cade (centre) and other staff members discuss patient care at a staff conference at Royal Park Mental Hospital, undated.
(Photographer unknown)

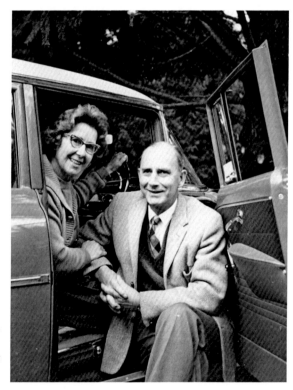

Jean and John Cade,
c. 1960s.
(Image courtesy of
Cade family)

20

On the day of the coronial inquest, the weather forecast was for a depression over south-eastern Australia, and John could have been forgiven for thinking he was smack-bang in the middle of it. By the time he travelled to the city morgue to present his account of his clinical care of the dead man, John, we can imagine, was nervy, replaying his version of events over and over. John knew he'd dabbled with a novel medicine, a crude and untested treatment. He himself had imbibed lithium, drinking it, secretly, in isolation. Dozens of guinea pigs were injected with it; they, for the most part, were buried deep beneath the grounds of a mental hospital. By today's standards, none of this was adequate preparation for using lithium on a suffering human being. But in circumstances where other therapies had proven ineffective, John proceeded to prescribe lithium. Now his first patient, Bill Brand, was also dead, and the reasons for this were about to be delved into publicly. Although some of his patients on lithium seemed to thrive, John must have been sensitive to the potential for public scandal and professional disgrace. This was the situation he faced when he sat before the hard-headed coroner in the Melbourne morgue that October day.

Given his predicament, it is only natural to ask how a man might react in such a tight spot. Would he try to manipulate the evidence, or, if desperate enough, even falsify it? Would he do anything to point the bone away from himself? More likely, he'd do the very human thing we all employ in moments of self-preservation—subtly shift the emphasis here and there to present ourselves in the best possible light. Perhaps, if John was a treacherous man, he might shed blame entirely on to someone or something else. So how, in this very uncomfortable moment, did John Cade respond to the Coroner's interrogation?

What he did was what we might have hoped for in a man who lived life with stone-edged integrity. If John felt giddy as he prepared for the coroner, his notes do not reveal it. Rather, he settled the commotion in his mind, and responded to the cross-examination with a taut, one-page synopsis of Bill Brand's medical history. John's characteristic steady script—concise and without any hint of deception—told how he had prescribed lithium for Bill; that it resulted in remarkable improvement, but was discontinued due to side effects. He did not embroider the truth; he did not gloss over any anomaly or justify his actions. There is not a crooked sentence or a contorted syllable in his deposition. It was as clean-cut as the man himself. If John were an artist, he'd be a minimalist; embellishment was never his game. A less scrupulous man may have been tempted to fudge the cause of death, or at least to limit the guilt attributed to lithium. John did nothing of the sort. When it came to his opinion as to the cause of death he squared up to his responsibilities and wrote with the certainty of biblical authority (and presumably his God watched over his shoulder) that death was due to the combined effects of lithium toxicity, starvation and chronic mania. No flinching, no excuses. You could not have asked for a more brutally honest response in a situation where a man might have been seduced into deception. If nothing else, John Cade showed himself to be a man of unquestionable probity.

When his son Jack reflected on his father's deposition, there was no surprise: 'My father was a very proper person . . . if he had a legal concern he would have put it straight, not shillyshallied around, or hiding anything. He was always very upfront on those things.'

A patient's death means a lot to a doctor, especially when that doctor's treatment caused the death. Even more so when that treatment is bravely or perhaps recklessly plucked from nowhere. None of us, unless we have power over life and death, can truly comprehend the emotions that coursed through John's mind, but there is little doubt that he was profoundly wounded by the death of Bill Brand. Whatever troubling thoughts John held about Bill's death, they remained captive within his breast, and were never shared with friends, family or colleagues. It might be said that sometimes the impact on a doctor is measured not by how often he talks about a patient's death but, rather, how he seeks to avoid it, and John, in all his subsequent writings, never penned a further word about the death of the first man he treated with lithium.

While John pondered the death of Bill Brand, on the other side of the world and seemingly unbeknown to John, lithium was under scrutiny.

The problem started innocently enough—with table salt. The same salt we nonchalantly and typically in excess sprinkle on our fish and chips, the salt we taste on our tongues every time we take a dip in the ocean. Indeed, this salt can be found just about everywhere. And everyone knows that table salt, chemically speaking, is sodium chloride.

Table salt was about to play an important role in the history of lithium and mental illness. By the late 1940s, patients who suffered from high blood pressure were advised to cut their consumption of salt. Reducing salt intake cuts blood pressure and eases the burden on the heart as the heart pumps blood around the body. So around the world, patients with hypertension were placed on low-salt diets. These diets, if you've ever been condemned to try them, are pretty bland to the taste. In the United States—where every consumer-driven niche is a commercial opportunity—alert companies scanned about for an alternative to table salt: something that would give a flavour-some taste to food but wouldn't increase blood pressure. Any solution to this problem would rake in millions of dollars; American capitalism found this solution without drawing breath.

Soon, at least four different American companies believed they'd struck a savoury bonanza. While experimenting with alternatives to table salt they came across lithium, discovering that if you replaced sodium with lithium in table salt you produced a substance that also has a salty taste—lithium chloride. The solution seemed obvious: instead of sodium chloride on your fish and chips, just lavish lithium chloride on it. The taste would rejuvenate the dullest of diets, and, importantly, there would be no damage to your heart or rise in blood pressure. Lithium chloride was marketed in the United States under proprietary names such as Foodsal and Westsal. Post-war affluent America, with its ample and ever-expanding middle-class girth, could shovel in this new salt by the tonne.

It all seemed innocuous enough. That is, until things started to go terribly wrong.

In March, 1949—a year after John started his experimental lithium treatment of Bill Brand—four research papers were published in *The Journal of the American Medical Association*: each paper suggested that lithium was a poison. The ominous research told the stories of sixteen patients, all of whom showered the salt substitute—lithium chloride—on their food. These articles make for graphic reading. Patients started to shake and were rendered incapable of holding a knife and fork; others dissolved into convulsions, and some staggered about, unable to find their balance. A few slurred their words before collapsing into a coma. Three died; others nearly did so, but clung to life after heroic medical measures. Lithium in each and every case was dangled as the culprit.

A news flash from Chicago listed four deaths from lithium. These were the above deaths, plus one other, and they warned of more to come.

Further news of lithium's toxicity swarmed through the US medical community, and, before long, the entire nation knew of it. In one blow, lithium was a name virtually no American wanted to be associated with: no doctor, no patient and certainly no politician.

The political response was fearsome and swift; federal agents rummaged through pharmacies and warehouses clearing out supplies. *The New York Times* reported that 40 health inspectors scoured over 4000 pharmacies and over 400 health food shops.

New York City's Commissioner of Health, Dr Harry S. Mustard—sporting an impeccably correct name for a food crisis—warned and 'appealed to all persons having lithium chloride salts to destroy them at once'.

Time magazine chimed in and broadcast to the nation the US Food and Drug Administration's directive: 'Stop using this dangerous poison at once.' Newspapers from Chicago to New York to Arizona ran articles alerting the population and advising doctors. All was confusion, except on one point of certainty: all fingers pointed at lithium.

Lithium was rooted out from pharmacies, health shops and warehouses and—most of all—from the American diet.

And, of course, being the United States, following this national delirium of fear there threatened a furious flood of lawsuits. In a flash, lithium was gone.

But in all of this monumental mayhem, one question was trampled upon and rarely asked: Why was lithium, this savoury substitute the Americans were contorting themselves to banish, so readily available in the United States anyway? If it was poisonous, how was it already so freely available in the marketplace?

The answer, it turns out, is that lithium, in one form or other, had long been in the American diet. Lithium was not regarded as a drug, but as a health-promoting dietary supplement. This meant that in the 1940s Americans didn't need a doctor's prescription to get lithium; all they had to do was to walk into a health food store and simply ask for it. And its presence in the American diet goes well back, at least to the nineteenth century. Lithium spilled into the New World from the nineteenth-century drawing rooms of Victorian England, where it had been lauded for its supposed magical healing powers and as a general 'pick-me-up' tonic for many years. But it was in the United States that lithium secured its strongest commercial foothold; during the late nineteenth and early twentieth century, lithium was consumed in a manner scarcely believable.

It all started with the bottling and selling of naturally occurring mineral waters, riding upon the back of natural springs around the world. Then, of all things, came lithium beer, brewed and marketed in Wisconsin; and in 1929, in the weeks before Wall Street crashed, the popular soda drink, 7-Up, was launched, boasting lithium as an ingredient. The truth is, lithium was plentiful in the American diet by the 1940s; it's just that most people didn't know it; and, more importantly, no one was dying from it.

Only when lithium chloride—marketed as a salt substitute for cardiac patients—was swallowed in vast amounts did its toxicity surface. That's when people died and everyone took notice. So in 1949 when a shrill *New York Times* shrieked that lithium was 'a dangerous poison' and had killed four people; and that 'more deadly salt' had been safely sequestered, it was as if toxic waste from a nuclear test zone was contaminating the nation's food bowl. There was nowhere for lithium in the United States to go—other than oblivion. And that is where it duly went.

It would be over twenty years before lithium was reintroduced to the United States as a medical therapy. Meanwhile, Australia's isolation in the 1950s would serve lithium well. For in Melbourne, nearly 13,000 kilometres from the United States, lithium lingered in the back wards of a handful of psychiatric hospitals. All it needed was a doctor willing to use it . . .

21

Forces gathered to pulverise lithium back into the earth's crust, not only in the United States, as we have seen, but also back home in Australia. Within weeks of John's lithium paper coming out in *The Medical Journal of Australia*, a note by John appeared as a loose insertion in another publication, the newsletter sent to psychiatrists in Australia four times a year.

It is not hard to imagine that a man who introduces a novel and potentially brilliant treatment might have his detractors as well as his admirers. And in this relatively small circle of competitive Australian psychiatrists, John could count both. The insertion records John asking his fellow psychiatrists that, if they used lithium, could they monitor patients for toxic effects and pass any observations back to him. It was a prudent and, we suspect, a slightly worried communication. There is no doubt that while John savoured the idea of lithium's promise, the reported deaths and then the banning of lithium in the United States left him wavering, anxious as to the outcome of further treatments.

If John was at all worried that no Australian doctor would take up lithium, he need not have been. Australia doctors embraced it with extraordinary gusto. Within a year of John's paper, well over a hundred (perhaps over 200) patients were on lithium around Australia. From Melbourne to Perth to Sydney and back to Melbourne, solutions of lithium were being stirred, shaken and poured. Most of these were prepared in the chain of mental asylums that stretched around the country, but there were also private psychiatrists coming on board. This was a medical world hungry for new treatments and lithium was a glimmer of hope that enticingly stretched before doctors and patients. If it could be shown to work consistently and safely, it would revolutionise the care of the mentally ill. But, as John knew, it was not without possible mortal cost. One such cost, of course, was the death of Bill Brand. The coroner had concluded that death was from 'broncho-pneumonia following upon lithium poisoning, consequent upon treatment with lithium salts, which the state of health of deceased warranted'.

Although Australia is a vast land, the psychiatric community in the 1950s was little more than a hundred strong and, like juicy gossip in a small town, news of deaths from an experimental treatment didn't take long to sweep through to every psychiatrist. It turned out that Bill Brand's death was not the first from lithium. John must have known of the other two lithium deaths before his own patient, Bill, died. One perished in the Victorian country town of Ballarat, the other in Perth, on the other side of the nation.

The town of Ballarat rose, spectacularly, from the gold discoveries of the 1850s, when Victoria was one of the wealthiest places on the planet. A rural centre with nearly 50,000 residents in 1950, the town had contracted from its glorious past. A two-hour drive west from Melbourne, its sprawling 83-hectare asylum for the mentally ill was a vast repository for psychiatric patients, which, at its peak, housed close to a thousand inmates. Constructed in 1869 as the Ballarat Industrial School, its building stock was overhauled in the late 1930s. By the early 1950s a visitor to the mishmash of old and new buildings remarked upon how 'birds rested in the ward ceilings' and how their droppings constantly 'fouled the beds' in which patients slept. Most wards were locked, straitjackets commonplace and windows barred. Remembered for the bitter and biting breezes that skipped in from the waters of nearby Lake Wendouree, patients kept warm by polishing the floors with beeswax and huddling about coal fires in open hearths.

At Ballarat, a single doctor might attend over 300 patients, making it impossible to offer any kind of meaningful medical care, let alone understanding each man's or woman's needs. Indeed this was hardly expected. The doctor who piques our interest was Dr 'Nick' (Edgar) Roberts, a stocky, affable man who, in a photo taken some years later, is pictured at the Ballarat Mental Hospital rugged up in thick layers topped by a woollen scarf and sporting a broad-broom moustache: the spitting image of a British sergeant-major.

Among the throng of human flesh under the care of Dr Roberts was one Mary Niblett, in her late 50s, whose occupation was listed as home duties, though she'd not had a house to clean for the four years since her admission to the asylum. Mary was, at least according to the staff, a terrier of a patient—violent, aggressive and noisy, petulant and demanding, 'constantly maniacal for the past three years'. With not a hint of her hurricane abating, she was a superb candidate for an experimental treatment. Nick Roberts had read John's lithium paper—there was probably no Australian psychiatrist who hadn't—and followed John's treatment protocol to the chemical letter. And so Mary was started on a solution of lithium citrate on 19 December 1949. To improve its palatability, a sweetener called 'syrup of orange' was added, a common asylum trick to entice patients to take medicine. Nursing staff were then given a crisply typed list of toxic lithium symptoms to watch for. One week later, on lithium, Mary was placid and seemingly on the mend. But it was a deceptive calm. A day later she fell ill—clutching her abdomen and vomiting—and could hardly hold a straight line as she walked. Lithium was ceased, but to no avail. Seizures rapidly followed; coma consumed her. Two days later Mary Niblett was dead, the first Australian patient to die from lithium toxicity.

Dr Roberts wrote up the case in a report he submitted to *The Medical Journal of Australia* as a warning to other doctors, and, with a sharp mind, suggested that an effective dose of lithium for mania may be too close to the toxic dose. His paper urged doctors to use caution if prescribing lithium.

———

The second patient to die from lithium toxicity was Frank Kyd. A former orchardist, Kyd had been in mental hospitals, on the other side of the continent, in Western Australia, for fifteen years; when manic he went on wild and destructive rampages before collapsing into fitful sleeps. After an initial improvement on lithium, Kyd lapsed into the now familiar constellation of toxicity: he was confused, slurred his speech and lurched about like a drunkard at closing time. Shortly afterwards, the nurses could not rouse him. Death soon followed.

Kyd's doctor was Bernard Glesinger, an immigrant doctor with an MD from Vienna, who, like Nick Roberts in Ballarat, had read John's paper and dispensed lithium with an astonishing speed. Within months, Glesinger was pouring lithium into over a hundred patients at Claremont Mental Hospital in Perth. Most did well; only Kyd died. A post-mortem was conducted, but there was no coroner's inquest. The post-mortem, dealing only with an examination of the body and not with the effects of treatment, was unable to determine the cause of death. That was left to Glesinger, who concluded that lithium toxicity was to blame.

Frank Kyd died some 2700 kilometres away from Melbourne. Perth—famously parochial and prosperous—is the most isolated city in the most isolated continent on earth. In 1950, when cost and travel time to Perth made it inaccessible to most Australians, Perth could very well have been Timbuktu to those living in Melbourne. Digging metals out of the ground was to become Perth's passport to prosperity in the twentieth century, but at Claremont Mental Hospital only one metal—lithium—was drawing attention.

Aspects of what took place at Claremont tell us something about how and why lithium was widely used in Australia at this time. The superintendent was Frank Prendergast, one of John

Cade's closest chums, a fellow alumnus from his university days. It was probably no coincidence that lithium was being used so extensively at Claremont, as John and Frank were in regular contact. But it was a difficult time for Prendergast—a royal commission into 'cruelty allegations against certain male attendants at the Claremont Mental Hospital' was under way. And this investigation raised something of interest to us: lithium. It came to light that a ten-year-old boy, 'a notorious juvenile' as reported by a journalist in *The West Australian*, was detained in the hospital. The boy's treatment included 'electric shock and lithium'. It seems, if this report is accurate, that just about any patient was fair game for lithium. John Cade, of course, had no control on how lithium might be used in hospitals around Australia. But, if he'd had any inkling of lithium's questionable use in a child, we can only imagine it would have kindled his nervousness.

By the time Bill Brand was stretched out on a cold slab in a Melbourne morgue, the rollcall of lithium deaths stood at three. It remains unclear whether this number was an accurate count of deaths caused by lithium at that time. Whereas Victorian law required that every unexpected death in a mental hospital go to the coroner for investigation, this was not the case in every state. The late 1940s and early 1950s was a different age, in which activities in mental hospitals were not under the same scrutiny as today. If three lithium deaths occurred in modern Australian hospitals, it would likely provoke an army of investigative journalists, tell-all documentaries, and a bevy of whistle-blowers. None of this occurred and the early 1950s allowed lithium to survive in the mental hospitals of Australia. Moreover, as a counter to these occasional negative reports on lithium, there were positive medical publications and encouraging clinical observations that fostered enthusiasm for its use.

One such example of a positive report came from Sunbury Mental Asylum, on the northern outskirts of Melbourne, where John had lived as a primary-school student back in 1922. Val

Ashburner, a psychiatrist at Sunbury, enthused over lithium, finding it such an irresistible option that he siphoned the solution out with stunning results. Twelve of the more than 50 patients to whom he prescribed lithium were liberated of all signs of illness, striding out of the asylum and into the community; none died. So zealous was Ashburner that—like a small outback mining town—the Sunbury hospital pumped no less than 15 pounds (7 kilograms) of the metallic lithium crystal into patients, grain by tiny grain, in rapid time.

So what did John make of these emerging and highly divergent reports on lithium? There were some remarkable successes mixed with occasional appalling and ugly deaths. Patients were in need of care, but what care was appropriate? Was it reasonable to experiment with lithium when it might eventually harm or kill the patient, even though the result might be remarkably positive for the patient in the short term? In the midst of these questions there was a sense that metropolitan and regional coroners, along with mental hospital doctors and administrators, agreed without saying as much that an experiment was in progress, and was justified. Six decades later, we are left to ponder precisely what John made of it all because, frustratingly, he left behind no personal notes from this time about lithium. Later in his life, when asked about this period he didn't divulge a great deal, and kept whatever hopes and misgivings he had to himself. So it is with a paucity of such intimate information we fossick through newspapers, peruse private letters, and try to unpick and interpret behaviours and beliefs played out over 60 years ago.

John, we might speculate, was hopeful about lithium's future, but it is clear he harboured doubts, even a foreboding, about how it all might end. And along with this undertow of doubt, John was also aware of the many potential critics around him, circling. But mostly there was still an air of curiosity about lithium—had something truly remarkable been unearthed, or, as is so often the case in the history of psychiatry, would it prove to be just another dud and dangerous treatment?

So, unlike the Americans, who had abandoned lithium, John did not totally toss out his fascination with this soft, white metal. Instead he waited, while lithium's impact was weighed for better or for worse.

22

In some quarters, John's lithium discovery was seen as just the thing to try to lever the medieval world of psychiatry into the modern penicillin-age of medicine. And for that initiative there were rewards. Medicine, like the military, offers recognition through rank; discipline and chain of command are deeply embedded in both. Just as rising from captain to major was an elevation for John during the war, so in parallel was the elevation from psychiatrist to superintendent in the world of the asylum. In late 1950, almost certainly because of his lithium research, John was promoted to the position of medical superintendent at Bundoora Mental Hospital.

Although he was a man who frowned upon ostentation and public brouhaha about achievements, John was privately pleased with his ascension. David, his second boy, remembers one particular day at primary school after this promotion when all the children were asked about their father's occupations: 'I told everyone my dad was a doctor. I thought that was pretty good. But when I got home and told dad, he said I should have said, "Psychiatrist superintendent of Bundoora Mental Hospital" instead of doctor. He was proud of that.'

But the clearest evidence we have that his lithium work had drawn favourable attention came when John was invited to deliver two public lectures on psychiatry at the University of Melbourne. Known as the Beattie Smith lectures, this was an outstanding distinction for a young psychiatrist, and it placed his name before the general public. From that point onwards, the name John Cade was a staple in the Melbourne media.

The brace of Beattie Smith lectures—an annual public event in the city of Melbourne's calendar—was delivered by a distinguished psychiatrist in an effort to advance the treatment of mental illness. The lectures were named after William Beattie Smith, an English psychiatrist who had migrated to Australia in the 1880s. John's father remembered Beattie Smith, describing him as a good-looking man of trim build with a closely clipped beard. Soon after arrival, Beattie Smith made Australia home and found work at the Ararat Lunatic Asylum. He proved a man of unconventional turn, who, in addition to his drive to improve medical teaching, insisted that attendants undertake the apparently revolutionary act of wearing uniforms. In his spare time he tilled the arable Ararat soil into a vineyard, which remains today testimony to a fertile and varied mind. At his death, unmarried and wealthy, he bequeathed 1000 pounds for his eponymous annual lectures to be held at the University of Melbourne. So, as announced in *The Argus* in May 1951, Dr John Cade, medical superintendent of Bundoora Repatriation Hospital, would step onto the podium at the University of Melbourne's medical school to deliver his first well-prepared public oration. Overnight, John was catapulted into the limelight.

John was not a man to reveal his inner qualms, never a 'gossip or blabbermouth' as Jean so quaintly put it, least of all about what orbited in his own brain. But he was nervous leading up to his first Beattie Smith lecture. This surprised his family, for within the Cade household his equanimity under pressure was legendary. Jean remembered how on one occasion, her husband was speaking before an all-female audience, when partway through his speech John realised that his fly was undone. Without skipping a verbal beat, and in full view of his admiring audience, John casually zipped up his fly, apologised *en passant*, and continued on imperturbably. Jean remembered his, as always, meticulous preparation in the dining room at their Bundoora home, standing rigidly upright in a corner and rehearsing to his imagined audience, and running through the many iterations to get his words just right:

I knew he was nervous. So was I. The Beattie Smith lecture . . . was a great honour. John was very exercised in his mind [as to] how he could make it interesting to all the colleagues who would come and yet for the public to enjoy it and understand it.

He always read them to me. If he was going to stand on a platform he practised standing in the corner of a room and I listened without interrupting. I had listened to his speech many times at home . . . and I would tell him how it felt and how he looked.

When John arrived at the university's medical school on the evening of 7 May to deliver the first of two lectures, Jean sat in the front row of the steeply tiered wooden seats—presumably casting a furtive flick of her eyes over her husband's fly to ensure all was well secured. The university boasts the oldest functioning medical school in the nation. And the old anatomy lecture theatre, over the century, was home to thousands of note-taking students as white-coated prosectors displayed human anatomical specimens for viewing. But on this night it was a psychiatrist on centre stage, and John would take apart the human mind for display. Jean recalled: 'The place was packed.'

When introduced, John, dry mouthed, rose to speak. In his habitual style, he looked out over the array of heads before him, not focusing on any one person, and replicated what he'd done so often before with Jean in their Bundoora dining room. In the crammed theatre, journalists from the Melbourne press positioned themselves to take notes on the latest developments in psychiatry. They sensed a revolution in the making.

John knew some of what he was about to say would ruffle his colleagues and, perhaps, damage his own future. It didn't matter; he'd speak his mind as he always did. John, gently spoken and clear-minded, drew his sketch of psychiatry as he saw it. He spoke with a fastidious care for words and a love of history. And as he did so, nervousness gave way to unaffected self-assurance. His words rolled out across the auditorium.

Over the two evenings, a week apart—as reported in the Melbourne newspapers—John ranged across the different fields of psychiatry. But there was one acerbic comment for which John is still most remembered. It was a rebuke of what he saw as a backward step in psychiatry—Sigmund Freud and his ther-apies: 'I believe that Freudian psychology has cast a blight upon the minds of men that will last perhaps another 50 years. I can see the hackles of most of my colleagues visibly rising . . .' Freud was all the rage across the psychiatric world and John Cade knew it. Nonetheless he took aim with his carefully sharpened harpoon and boldly fired at Freud. This was a stirrer's provocation to roil his fellow psychiatrists.

Watching his colleagues—drawing their collective breath of indignation and hemmed in by their tiny timber seats in the anatomy theatre—we can only imagine that John, from his podium perch, was almost enjoying the moment.

When interviewed 50 years later, Jean remembered this precise moment in her husband's speech with exceptional freshness, and, in whispered tones, she went on that no one applauded what many regarded as blasphemy. In preparing her husband beforehand, and sensing the likely disapproval of his colleagues, she counselled John about criticising Sigmund Freud: 'You can't say that about

[Freud], he's the darling. Why don't you just not mention him . . . But that was John.' The real issue here was that John pushed hard the notion that serious psychiatric illnesses should be seen like any other medical illness; that its root cause was an underlying physical problem within the brain. But the very idea that illnesses such as mania or schizophrenia were the result of an abnormal Periodic Table of the brain was beyond many of his colleagues. They couldn't stomach the notion that chemistry lay at the heart of this human behaviour. This was the battle John faced.

Some of his colleagues were visibly affronted, their contempt plain, refusing to applaud. But it seems the general public and the press lapped it up. John spoke to them in a language so sensible, so down-to-earth, that just for a moment, psychiatry made beautiful sense, leaving in the common person's mind an image of psychiatry as sturdy, testable, without a hint of gibberish.

John Cade possessed, in particular, one rare and remarkable quality. He was wonderfully free of the fear of what his colleagues might think of him—an unusual quality in a doctor, perhaps an unusual quality in anyone. He was never encumbered by the craven need to look good before his fellow doctors. This liberated him to say things others would not. Best of all, he could not resist poking fun at the pomposity of his own profession. Take the Beattie Smith oration, for example. At one point in his oration John critiqued the then widely held, but absurd, belief that schizophrenia was caused by faulty parental upbringing. If this were indeed true, John went on, it would be preventable by an upbringing in a family with 'healthy habits of mind'. And then, as a barb to his all-too-smug colleagues, he said, 'but I may remark in passing that the offspring of psychologists and psychiatrists have not yet achieved a reputation for outstanding stability'. We have no record of how this was received by the psychiatrists in his audience, but we can imagine John bore a deep inner grin as the words left his lips.

The Beattie Smith lectures gave John a chance to talk to the world, or at least to Melbourne, about his recent lithium discovery.

But the word lithium never breached his lips. Surely he was tempted to tell a wider audience about lithium? But he chose not to. So what was going on in John's mind? Was he so apprehensive about lithium's safety that he chose to hold his fire? Or was it a touch of humility? The answer, it seems, might have been a bit of both.

In his oration he does leave us an allusive clue about how he hoped lithium might prove its worth. He may not have articulated the word 'lithium', but everything about the words below points to his discovery of lithium as a treatment for mania:

> My qualifications for discussing medical research in general or even psychiatric research in particular are best left unstated. I might most kindly describe myself as an enthusiastic amateur, full of curiosity, with fair determination, golden opportunities, inadequate knowledge and woeful technique. But even the small boy, fishing after school in a muddy pond with string and bent pin, occasionally hauls forth a handsome fish ... Even more important, perhaps, is the determination to use any and every means to the end, no matter how humble, how unorthodox or how tedious.

When John questioned his own ability as a researcher, we can take it that this was not false modesty. Even his most ardent supporter, his wife, was happy to depose that John was 'not even a researcher's bootlace', although we might suspect that she was quoting John himself in one of his more humorous and gently self-deprecating moments.

There is one further memory of John's oration, one that is not filed in the archives of oblivion in a State Library or printed in a 1951 broadsheet. Russell Meares, an eminent professor of psychiatry, recalls how his father, Ainslie Meares, also a psychiatrist, heard and remembered John's speech. Ainslie Meares knew John Cade well. Indeed Ainslie was one of the few private psychiatrists who bothered to turn up for the regular quarterly educational meetings of a newly formed group of public hospital psychiatrists. Most psychiatrists who worked in private practice refrained from attending, regarding public-hospital psychiatrists as being of a lower station. When Ainslie turned up at these meetings as the lone private psychiatrist, he did so in grand style, pulling up in his Rolls-Royce.

Russell Meares recalled his father's comments on John's Beattie Smith oration:

> My father remembers John Cade, and his rather unusual statements about Freud. He told me that the psychiatrists in the audience looked upwards, towards the ceiling; embarrassed, they groaned and smirked a bit and covered their mouths with their hands, as if somehow trying to expel the distaste of the criticism of Freud. My father put it down to Cade's Catholicism.

John Cade never flaunted his Catholicism—by nature he was disinclined to be demonstrative about anything; that was just not him. But neither could it be said that the social climate in Melbourne was conducive to revealing one's Catholic faith in public.

This was a time in Melbourne of mutual suspicion between Catholics and non-Catholics. Older Melburnians remember how it was not uncommon, for example, to find two adjacent local schools—one Catholic and one state school—where one started the day 15 minutes earlier than the other, just so Catholic and non-Catholic children didn't mingle as they walked, ran or hopped into their respective schoolyards, lest one faith tainted the other or fisticuffs broke out.

Eric Seal, a Catholic and a psychiatrist, recalls those bigoted days: 'When I entered Psychiatry in the early 1950s, I was regarded with some disfavour by many Catholics for being a psychiatrist, and by most psychiatrists for being a Catholic.' It was perhaps a touch of self-protective wisdom that kept John quiet about the deepest of his beliefs.

The Catholic Church of the 1950s was ill at ease with psychiatry: uneasy about the way psychiatry sought to unravel and explain human behaviour; uneasy that psychiatry had no need for sin or to call for a higher power. And of all the types of psychiatry, the Freudian world of bestial impulse and sexual desire seemed the most godless of all. The Catholic fear was that Freudian ideas might undermine and usurp the Catholic way of understanding humanity. John Cade was a rising medical star, one the Catholic Church could ill-afford to let go. The Church saw John as a means of exerting influence in psychiatry, and approached him.

Deeply religious, John attended church on Sunday with the precision of an atomic clock. In John Cade, the Catholic Church had a man who was not only a young prominent psychiatrist, but one who espoused an understanding of mental illness that was more acceptable to the church: that mental illness should be seen as a branch of medicine with a chemical basis to disorders, not some jiggery-pokery world of Freudian fantasies.

As a result John was invited to write a monthly article for a national Jesuit magazine, *The Messenger*. The first of these was published on 1 September 1951. John went by the nom de plume, 'Mensana', meaning 'sound in mind', and if the editorial comments are to be believed, his articles were a smashing success with Melbourne's Catholics. John's articles offered common-sense advice on anything from juvenile delinquency, to anxious children, to the elderly with dementia.

John wrote, unapologetically, that the soul and spiritual belief were as central to mental health as any techniques employed by psychiatrists. In response to the question of how to raise children as cocksure Catholics in the modern world, John comes out swinging hard:

I'd sooner a child were brought up by good Catholic parents, who had not read one paragraph in press or magazines on how to bring up their children than by the most learned psychiatrist whose approach was governed solely by the findings of modern secular psychology.

In John Cade the church had a psychiatrist with a Catholic lining, a distinct and ecclesiastical elevation over a godless psychiatry.

23

Summer in January means one thing in Australia—holidays. And for the Cade family, like many Australians, it meant an annual pilgrimage to the beach. The Cades, with John at the helm, set forth every January in the early fifties to their favoured destination—the Kennett River. The campsite was on the coast just over 165 kilometres west of Melbourne.

Each holiday John would pack the car (a Chevrolet having replaced the Dodge by the start of the 1950s), attach the caravan sitting in the backyard, and Jean, Jack, David, and the two younger Cades—Peter and Richard, born since the tragic death of Mary—would pile in. As they rumbled down the road from their house through the mental hospital, the patients would line up to watch their superintendent take off for a month.

The Cades and their caravan travelled along the Great Ocean Road, which hugs one of the world's most picturesque coastlines. Dug out of the cliff face, some of it by hand by returned First World War soldiers needing employment, the road is dedicated to those who perished in that conflict. It stands, according to tourism brochures, as the world's biggest war memorial. But in the early 1950s it was less than flash and was what one might have expected in a time of post-war austerity—narrow, winding and inordinately dangerous in parts as heavy vehicles squeezed past in opposing directions.

On arriving at Kennett River, Jean, John and the boys would catapult out of the car and dash to the beach, where the southern currents deep from the Antarctic brought chilled water to this Victorian coastline. Carved blue curls hit the rocks with a steady pulse that John would have admired. Jean remembers spending hours basking on a beach towel while John, like a mischievous seal, swam and gambolled in the waves. Their first year at the Kennett was in 1950. John adored its location so much that they soon purchased a house in the vicinity and ditched the caravan.

In the first few years at the Kennett, John and the two older boys learned the art of body surfing from a local instructress, whom the boys remember as 'built like a large beach ball on legs', and they got to know the handful of other regular holiday visitors. There was always something to see, and not all of it related to the picture-book beauty of the coastline. While not quite Changi, the art of conserving anything of value at the Kennett was ever-present, and the boys recollect John taking great pride in showing them the value of wise water use:

> The drinking water was tank water, collected from roof run off . . . There was only a 500 gallon tank in the roof so there was none to spare for showering. Dad showed us how, when he was a POW, he had learnt to manage his morning ablutions with just an enamel mug of warm water. First he would clean his teeth; then he would wet his face and lather up and shave; then wet a flannel and soap his face and 'APC' (armpit and crutch) then rinse with the residual water from the mug. Of course, he'd boil the large kettle for Mum to have a more civilised wash.

At the Kennett, John often withdrew into himself and struck out on long nature walks, combing the beach or exploring the abutting Otway Ranges, observing and listening in a manner that fed on the stillness about him. Deep from the belly of the ocean, the baritone rumble of the southern seas was the backdrop to all his wanderings.

He observed and noted the geology of the rocks and the stories they told, and played in the surf, tasting the salt of the water upon his tongue as the sea foamed over his body like vintage champagne. On his haunches, John might trace a line of seaweed, or follow the meandering beach trail of a sea snail; at night he'd hear the tide pulsing in and the suck of the ocean pulling it all back again. In this world of solitary strolls, and sealed from the intrusions of an insistent world, there was nothing to rupture his reverie.

The wilderness of the western Victorian coastline was a utopia for John. The Kennett River house had no electricity, no sewer, no water; the boys read by kerosene lamps and Jean cooked on a wood stove. Photographs of John's time here are revealing. Some of his stiffness of manner, and lack of spontaneity, were shed on the sands of the Kennett River. His smiles wreathe his face from ear to ear. We can't help but sense that this was where he was happiest.

———

Melbourne was a political and social powder keg in the early 1950s, with rivals fighting to gain acceptance for their ideas about Australia's future. Discord was rife within psychiatry, just as it was within the universities and within political parties. In 1948 and again in 1950, major reports slammed the administration and poor condition of Victorian mental hospitals, and John's mentor, the ageing Dr John Catarinich, was widely scapegoated.

Privately, Catarinich stood accused of trashing one of the cornerstones of Australian society—its secular, non-religious custom of employing public servants on their ability and aptitude, not on their religious beliefs. He was accused of favouring the employment and promotion of Catholic mental-health staff over those holding other beliefs. Little did anyone know that he was also surreptitiously attempting an even bigger heist—to woo Catholic students wanting a career in psychiatry away from the recently established postgraduate university education program. He promoted a Catholic teaching unit in psychiatry designed to foreground Catholic religious values and traditions over all others.

The impulse that drove Catarinich and his allies in this endeavour was fear of 'godless communism'. Communism had steadily gained ground in Europe, and closer to home—in China, Indochina, Malaya and Korea—after the Second World War. Taking a giant leap of logic, this group of psychiatrists conflated a godless communism with Freudian doctrines that interpreted a belief in God as childish nonsense. It goes without saying that Catarinich was right behind Prime Minister Menzies when he sought to ban the Communist Party in Australia in 1951 via a controversial referendum. This act by an authoritarian Menzies was incendiary and bitterly divisive; the referendum was defeated by a slender margin.

John Cade was a conservative in political matters, voting either for the Liberal Party or for the Catholic-dominated Democratic Labor Party, after its formation in 1955. Although he had concerns about communism, how he voted that referendum day is far from certain. But John had other, more immediate, matters to deal with. Things were changing rapidly. While Menzies' motion was in decline, John's trajectory was on the rise. His work on lithium and his Beattie Smith lectures pressed John's name forward; promotion was next. It was announced that he would move from Bundoora to take up the position of superintendent of Royal Park Mental Hospital in the heart of Melbourne, that city's only receiving house for newly diagnosed mentally ill men and women. It was a dramatic elevation in status and profile, and a telling affirmation of John's rising star.

As John prepared to leave Bundoora, his home for more than six years, the patients gathered as one and prepared to farewell him. Some high-minded psychiatrists might have dismissed Bundoora as a drowsy backwater, but John, who had made much of the opportunity to study and befriend its patients, felt at home there. His time at Bundoora continued a deep connection with the war and those tumbledown men who had suffered mental torment in battle.

John Cade, for his part, detested the war; he made no secret of that. And just as much, it seems, he abhorred any public show of emotion around its memory. He never joined the RSL; he never marched in unison with ex-soldiers on Anzac Day. He never joined the ex-serviceman who gambled their money in a game of two-up. It is likely that John saw this gambling game—a ring of ex-soldiers squawking over a couple of tossed coins like a mob of gulls around a hot chip—as a frivolous reminder of war. None of this was for John. What he did do was, privately and affectionately, meet the men of the 2/9th Field Ambulance to rekindle their kinship and refresh their bonds, drawn by a gravitational pull so powerful, outsiders were left to gaze and wonder. John cradled this extended army family close to his breast. They met, these men of the 2/9th, each year for an annual luncheon to dine on food and memories.

Some of the inmates at Bundoora Mental Hospital were members of the 2/9th, cobbers who'd been captured in Singapore. John's respect and love for these mentally crippled men was visible with every step he took on the grounds of the asylum. He spoke quietly with these men; there was nothing fancy about John. Nothing 'jammy, just plain ordinary', as Jean used to say.

Before her death in 2002, Jean Cade mused about these men, and their shared grief:

> When I go to the 2/9th luncheons . . . the men are so careful of their fellow man, so interested in them, they know about their families, about the ones who've died . . . quite a few women come, now they've lost their men. There is the most amazing brotherhood and I can say, love.

She recalled the sadness of uprooting her family from Bundoora, of packing their belongings in boxes, and the ascending affection of the mentally ill men for her husband as John prepared to leave:

> He loved his men at Bundoora. He really loved them and they loved him. They were all ex-servicemen. When we left we had

a nice dinner, but patients were there and they presented something to John. It was a moulded figure on a solid block. I think
it was pewter; a digger with his hat on with his knee up.

As John drew a veil over his time at Bundoora, and just five
days before he took up his new appointment at Royal Park, news
came through to him of an unexpected death at the Ararat Mental
Hospital, in northwest Victoria. Concetta Mollica, aged 49, was
one of thousands of Italians—fleeing poverty and fascism—who
had poured into Melbourne between the two world wars. Never
married, and with no relatives in sight, she'd been locked away in
asylums since 1929 when she was arrested for maliciously wounding
a Melbourne fruiterer with whom she'd had a dalliance. She'd been
an excitable and sometimes violent patient, and when electroconvulsive therapy failed to produce any improvement early in 1952, her
doctor resorted to lithium.

Her doctor at Ararat was Dr Nick Roberts, the very same
doctor who sounded the alarm about lithium after Mary Niblett
died early in 1950. That Roberts returned to the lithium well for
Concetta Mollica speaks to the desperation of doctors when they
reached the bottom of the bag of treatment options for the mentally
ill. It was now an inescapable fact: lithium could cure, but it could
also kill. It raised the stakes enormously. And this was lithium's
conundrum: in the face of thousands of tortured individuals who
might be resurrected from despair, should lithium be used, and if
so, how should it be used? Should doctors wait for the evidence to
mount in favour of a new treatment like lithium? Or should they
try a promising therapy in the full knowledge that the evidence
of benefit and how it actually worked was incomplete? Roberts
chose the latter approach, stating in a written submission to the
Coroner's Inquest, held soon after Concetta's death, that: 'She was
given not more than the dose [of lithium] found to have been safe
in many hundreds of patients who have been treated in this way in
many mental hospitals.'

Evidently lithium, despite its imperfections, was making a mark in the mental hospitals of Victoria. That aside, when Concetta Mollica's death was scrutinised, the coronial verdict was unambiguous: lithium toxicity.

24

In July 1952, John, Jean and their quartet of boys moved into their new home in Brunswick, a working-class suburb of Melbourne. The house spoke of past glory: a splendid Victorian manor, just outside the gates of Royal Park Mental Hospital, it was an imposing two-storey building with wrap-around verandahs, intricate cast-iron embellishments, a bay window and—as markers of a gentrified past—a maid's parlour, sewing room and stables out the back. A red brick courtyard in the rear, a garage and above it a hay loft, set off the property just nicely—the perfect home for John and his brood.

Inside, on the ground floor, included the dining room, John's expansive study, a large kitchen and scullery, a toilet, and, of all things, a 'flower' room, whatever that might be. One set of timber stairs led down to the depths of a cellar lined by bluestone walls; another set of stairs led upwards to the first floor, which had six bedrooms. From this floor, a further set of stairs led heavenwards to a lookout platform on the roof, where John could visit the stars and see the Melbourne skyline. Most rooms in the household had open fireplaces framed by marble and, as a remnant of a more leisured and socially stratified past, there were buttons in each room that summoned the domestic staff via a labelled signal box in the kitchen. The domestic staff were long gone by the time the Cades arrived.

Recently, over a thousand pounds had been spent on renovating the house for the new superintendent and his family. The estate was large, about an acre, and the garden impressive, and stood on the side of a hill that presided over the asylum and commanded views over much of Melbourne. It spoke of power and privilege; it was the natural position for the superintendent's house.

Brunswick, once the enclave of white Anglo-Saxon workers was in the 1950s a suburb undergoing serious demographic makeover. Post-war Melbourne saw a torrent of southern Europeans—especially Italians and Greeks—bulge through the Australian immigration sieve, the White Australia Policy. When the Cade children came to Brunswick they saw backyards all around them transformed into miniature vineyards thick with the pungent odour of fermenting grapes; creepers dangled from trellises as plots of land from Calabria were replicated in backyards across suburban Melbourne. Thousands of Mediterranean men in thick, heavy coats poured out of suburban trains after a day of grime in factories; middle-aged, round-faced women who uttered not a word of English roamed about in black dresses in a land that must have been as strange to them as they were to the Australians about them. These were the smells, the colours and the clothes, the culture of Brunswick, when John and his family arrived.

Inspired by the changes around him, it didn't take long for John to start his own garden filled with vegetables—sweet corn, asparagus, marrow and beans—and fruit trees, draped with a profusion of plums, apricots, nectarines and peaches, dropping their wares when ripe. John, hemmed in by the agriculture of southern Italy, even tried his hand at olive tree cultivation. And just like Bundoora, a dozen or so hens clucked about in the chook-house, offering the Cades fine, fresh eggs.

Royal Park was a very different hospital to Bundoora. Gone were the dairy cattle to milk, no acres of orchards brimmed with apples to pluck, and no drays meandered in tussocky paddocks for the Cade boys to ride; there was certainly less grassland to saunter about in taking pot shots at rabbits. The two older Cade boys—Jack and David—no longer forged intimate friendships with patients or entered into games in their imaginative worlds as they had once done at Bundoora. They, as much as their new hospital, had changed. Royal Park was bigger than Bundoora, but to these now older boys, it seemed smaller.

Royal Park, the most important psychiatric hospital in Melbourne, was a kind of central clearing house for the city's mentally ill. Opened in 1907, its original stated aim was to take in only those who had a reasonable chance of being cured of their affliction. But by 1952, all men and women who fell mentally ill in metropolitan Melbourne were sent for assessment to this one institution, and into its all-embracing arms came the alcoholics, the epileptics, the brain-injured, the manics, the depressives and every shade of mental affliction. Gone was the plodding lassitude of Bundoora; Royal Park was fast-paced and buzzed with life. It was the hub around which all of psychiatry in the state swirled. For the most part, Royal Park's aim was to treat people quickly and discharge them home. Those with incurable illnesses—such as the majority of people with schizophrenia—were shipped out to an archipelago of 'chronic' hospitals, like Beechworth and Sunbury, dotted around the city and the state. There, more likely than not, a patient would live out his or her natural life. Decisions that were made at Royal Park could determine the course of the rest of an individual's life.

John was 40 when he took up his appointment at Royal Park; in the conservative world of medicine, this was still a relatively young age for such an exalted position. John's speedy elevation to the crest of superintendent was not incremental but more as if he'd been flung from a catapult towards the heavens; not everyone was happy with such a rapid rise for the youngish doctor. It is little wonder that envious eyes tracked John Cade—a youthful-looking, springy squire of the manor—as he stepped into that role in 1952.

In the eyes of some, John was just a little too young, and a tad too inexperienced; and some of the aggrieved wives of psychiatrists, whose husbands had missed out on this plum post, weren't shy in letting people know of their dissatisfaction. This feminine disgruntlement came to the ears of John's wife, who heard of the whispered slurs accusing her husband of having 'jumped the queue'. Jean recalled: 'I remember a couple of the wives saying to me, "How did your husband get the post? Why did they favour John?"' Some designing wives were covert operatives for their men and ambitious for material gain and social status, even if their husbands were tardy about such distinctions. If sly words were daggers, Melbourne circa 1952 would have been awash with blood.

Two years before John Cade took up his appointment, the legislative framework for a spanking new government administration was set up to oversee mental health services in Victoria. It went by the slightly absurd name 'The Victorian Mental Hygiene Authority', terminology borrowed from the United States, implying that mental illness was a stain that needed cleansing. Well, if cleansing was needed, then fresh leadership was required to revamp and revitalise mental health services and break up the old cabal. Sadly—as was typical of the times in Australia—help was seen as coming from overseas, and overseas still meant one thing: England. That's how Dr Dax came to Australia.

Dr Eric Cunningham Dax was an imposing man of supreme erudition and lofty manner, of wide and passionate sensibilities, who drum-rolled his rrrr's, and confessed, on occasion, to being 'overbearing' to get the task done. He was just the man for the job. A princely Dax arrived in Melbourne in December 1951 to take up the chair of the newly created authority. With gusto, he set about the task of reforming a malnourished medical service.

Dax brought a breadth of interest and urgent intention that breathed life into a moribund mental health service. His psychiatric pedigree in England was varied; a master of craniometry—the craft of skull measurement—he once measured the head circumferences of 2000 severely mentally handicapped patients. And later, he worked on psychosurgery—treating mental illness by operating on the brain—helping to refine the size of the incision down to that of a five-cent piece.

And above and below and in between all of his medical work, Eric Cunningham Dax passionately collected Staffordshire China and pewter and adored fine music, all of which he innovatively brought to the banquet of ideas with which he was about to enrich Melbourne.

What Dax found in Melbourne's psychiatric asylums visibly distressed and shocked him: 'I remember well going to Kew [an institution for mentally disturbed children] and running my thumbnail down the wall; there was so much dirt and grease that a ridge was left behind.' On another occasion he recalled asking what the black colour on the tablecloth was, only to find that it was a thick swarm of flies. Among the many grotesque descriptions of grime, worn linoleum, cracked sewers and flaking paint, he remembered with detached English understatement that 'a good deal was done by improving the cleanliness and issuing toilet paper to avoid the drains being stopped up with newspaper'.

And what of Royal Park Hospital, John Cade's new domain? Well, in Dax's view it was little better, in fact, no better than 'a second-class boarding house and was quite unfit to receive early cases' of the mentally ill. John concurred with Dax on this point. But after a respectful beginning, theirs was a rocky relationship. John Cade, as the newly baptised superintendent of Royal Park, was to enjoy warm relationships over the years with many of his colleagues; Dr Dax was not one of them.

When John Cade took up his appointment at Royal Park he emphasised regular routines and the highest of clinical standards. Each morning John rose with the sun, consumed his customary breakfast of eggs and toast, smoked the first of his strategic cigarettes that marked out his day like the lines on a ruler, and drank his two piping hot cups of tea. He was on the wards by 8 am. He took the greatest of private pleasures in arriving on the wards before his junior doctors and reviewing the patients who had arrived during the night. The patients were often the fringe dwellers—the wanted and unwanted—of Melbourne, who walked the streets at night. Among them were the mentally ill, who stole into the darkness seeking safety and sustenance; others were criminals, usually of the petty type; still others were just homeless and lost. Many arrived unannounced at Royal Park; some were dragged in by the police, some by their families. Royal Park, at least, was a place of refuge for the night.

John Cade was not always comfortable in his role as medical superintendent. Indeed he often expressed his disdain for bureaucracy, for the minutiae of administration and its bloated and constipated rituals. He was first and foremost a clinician whose eyes sparkled in anticipation of a new patient. Not that he was a poor administrator; no one ever said that, but administration did not offer his fine brain the opportunities of detailed observation and deep reflection that clinical care so abundantly did. And as for research? John's new promotion meant that between his clinical and administrative duties there was little time for medical research. Despite this, John advocated that all psychiatrists should continue to question widely held beliefs on the cause and treatment of mental illness and undertake some sort of research. In his own assessment of his research capabilities, he still regarded himself as very much a novice in this field.

Jack and David recall being shown around the grounds of Royal Park by their father during these first few years. They still possess the most vivid recollections of watching electroconvulsive therapy, and roaming into the infamous padded cells where patients were isolated. 'The padded cells looked like a couch covered in leather and studded; the walls were also studded, all in a browny leather.' Straitjackets seemed more common here than at Bundoora, and were constructed of a coarse bone-coloured canvas: 'The sleeves had an extension on them that could be passed around the patient's waist, and tied just like a belt so that the arms were totally enclosed.' These were images of an era of asylum psychiatry that was about to fade, and fast.

At the end of each day John would leave his hospital office, stroll up the hill to his home and retire to his study, a luxury not offered at Bundoora. The study was an expansive wood-panelled room, and in winter there was an open fire framed by a rather ornate marble mantelpiece, flanked by bookshelves on either side. French windows looked out on to a gracious urban garden. John's library was a treasure and he read widely within and outside medicine: the shelves contained a complete set of Churchill's *A History of the English-speaking Peoples*; Gibbon's *The Decline and Fall of the Roman Empire*; mathematics and science texts; and Osler's *The Principles and Practice of Medicine*. Among them, almost forgotten among these hefty tomes, was the slim volume of Malay vocabulary from his Changi days. One could also find the evocatively titled gem *Rats, Lice and History*, in which John had underlined for attention: 'Yet, as everyone who has really been to war knows . . . it takes no time at all before the louse comes back to its own.' It's a safe bet that few psychiatrists were reading about the life and times of a louse. But then, John was never your average psychiatrist.

Although not embedded on the asylum grounds as they had been at Bundoora, the Cades still had their share of inquisitive patients who'd saunter up the hill to keep an eye on the new doctor. Jean remembers the 'occasional patient who came up and did some ironing; and we had a funny old fellow who dug around the garden'. Another patient or two would come for a cup of tea; John would give them cigarettes. 'They always called him Dr Cade.' Then there was psychotic Miss Ritchie, who entranced the Cade boys by sailing up and down the hill on her bicycle, which had a wire basket on its handle bars, carting things here and there, between hospital and house. Norman, a shrivelled-up man in a grey suit, worked in the woodshed; and then there was Doreen, the self-appointed house-maid for the Cades who—in the midst of her regular conversations with God—remembered with wonderful precision all the birthdays and anniversaries of John, Jean and the boys, and was a regular bearer of gifts for all the Cades.

The Cade household was one that bubbled with life; where hospital ended and home began was not always clear cut. And as for John's family, they were growing up: Jack and David were at Melbourne's prestigious Catholic boys school, Xavier College; Peter and Richard were at home, capering down to the hospital on tricycles or billy-carting down local streets, and attending primary school.

———

In 1952, the preferred treatment for the mental illness called schizophrenia was insulin coma therapy. And it is a therapy worth examining, to record and remember the types of care available to the mentally ill. Looking back, it seems preposterous that this treatment could have bloomed for so long and held such sway in the minds of psychiatrists. It was, simply put, a queer and at times hazardous treatment. But in the 1950s everyone, including John Cade, thought that insulin coma therapy was the gold-standard for schizophrenia, in the absence of anything more effective. And, like the hula hoop, insulin therapy for schizophrenia was a raging fad around the world. Every mental hospital that saw itself at the cutting edge of care had an insulin coma ward. At Royal Park, the insulin coma ritual started every Monday morning at 7 am on the dot, as the asylum grounds stirred to life.

At the appointed hour, about twenty or so young adult patients, all diagnosed with schizophrenia, were collected from around the hospital and ushered towards the insulin ward. Each patient was put into a bed and tucked tightly beneath a sheet; the blinds were drawn to darken the ward, and for the duration of the treatment no loud sounds were permitted. Next, a nurse pushing a trolley moved silently from bed to bed, injecting a small amount of insulin into each patient. Insulin, of course, lowers your blood glucose and, if you give enough, it makes you drowsy as your blood sugar falls. If you give a little more still, the patient drifts into coma. This was the desired treatment objective, with patients ideally experiencing one coma every day for at least a fortnight. One theory was that imposing this stress on the weak brain cells thought to be responsible for schizophrenia encouraged their destruction. Improvement rates varied wildly, somewhere between 20 and 50 per cent, though the statistical studies were fatally flawed by today's standards. Acceptance of these sorts of results by the psychiatric profession in the 1940s and 1950s, not to mention desperate families, underscores the hunger for any kind of treatment that offered even a glimmer of hope.

John Cade's son Jack volunteered as a nursing assistant during his school holidays. Part of his brief was to help give the insulin treatment, something we might now think inconceivable for a work-experience student. But his presence gives us a front-row seat. Jack remembers how, after the injections, sweat poured from the patients' pores and their skin glistened in the half-light; their faces drained of all colour until they were pasty and grey, and their breathing sank to a shallow and rapid flutter. For the next half an hour, the ward remained in this twilight state, patients softly breathing, nursing staff moving from bed to bed. From the end of the room it is not hard to imagine the scene: a line of bed-bound, linen-wrapped young men and women, pale heads poking above the sheets, eyes closed, wet hair pressed against their scalps.

Here and there one might see a patient wriggling like a worm beneath a sheet or hear an occasional moan crack the silence. Sometimes a full-blown epileptic convulsion (a side effect of the treatment) burst forth in one of the patients to snap the unnatural quiet of the room. But, for the most part, the room was filled with the soft sounds of rhythmic respiration.

Then, at a set time, John Cade or another one of the 'seniors' would instruct the nurses and junior doctors to bring the patients out of their soggy hibernation. To do so a tube was inserted via a patient's nostril and threaded down their oesophagus and into their stomach. A solution of glucose was sloshed down this tube to rapidly raise the person's blood glucose level and resurrect them into consciousness. Across the ward, figures would come to life, as though thawing out after a winter's deep freeze.

Very occasionally an individual patient did not move; that's when all hell broke loose on the ward. It is estimated that this treatment may have killed about one to five per cent of patients; many more were permanently brain damaged. These are rough figures, for only the scantiest of statistics were kept at the time. Older psychiatrists, who remember administering this treatment, recall it as the most terrifying experience of their careers.

The insulin coma treatment was repeated (although we might shudder at the thought) for each patient Monday to Friday, sometimes, for a period of up to twelve weeks. The deeply held belief was that in the afterglow of such treatment, delusions and hallucinations would vanish.

The following year, 1953, a paper was published in the British journal *The Lancet*, arguing that insulin coma therapy was not only dangerous but of no value at all. Within a decade it was a dead letter in Australian hospitals, and had vanished from any respectable hospital that purported to offer state-of-the-art care.

As far as we know, John did not undertake any further lithium research in his first year at Royal Park, but around Melbourne lithium was being used here and there, largely by individual psychiatrists who were keen to try it out. But its future was uncertain. It was at this point that a remarkable man emerged who changed everything, and who kept afloat John Cade's discovery.

25

Everyone who knew him, it seems, has a story about Eduard Michel Trautner. It is quite possible that lithium treatments would have died a natural death if it hadn't been for this exotic figure—a man who cut his medical research teeth in the drinking clubs of bawdy Berlin after the First World War; clubs where he researched the sex lives of flaxen-haired farm girls. At least, that's how the story goes. Or, more correctly, just one of the many stories about him. Everyone who knew him had a tale to tell; exotic and mischievous, and more than a little salacious, Eduard Michel Trautner, or as he was lovably called, Trautie, is the forgotten hero in the lithium story. Without Trautie the lithium story might well have trailed off into nothing.

A Bavarian Catholic by birth and atheist by choice, Eduard Trautner was a lance corporal in the German Army during the First World War; the story has it that he, lance raised, thundered on his stallion with the German cavalry into Belgium in the early days of the war. At war's end he studied medicine in Berlin and had a practice 'with the very rich and very eccentric'; he had a bent towards a study of sexuality and, according to one of his friends, took a particular interest in the study of homosexuality. Later in his life, Trautner enjoyed teasing his colleagues in Melbourne with his tales of the Weimar Republic's Berlin nightclubs and his clientele's libertine sexual behaviour. A radical man with the sniff of the dissident, by the early 1930s Trautner was a man on the run in Germany. Detesting Hitler and fearful of fascism, this very left-leaning doctor, it is speculated, was hunted out of Nazi Germany.

Rumour has it that he fled to Spain during the Spanish Civil War and ran a bar until he gathered together the exotic strands of his life and decamped to England. A man of many dimensions, he studied science including botany; one of his co-workers recalls Trautie vaguely saying something about working in a lab 'at either Cambridge or Oxford and marrying a daughter of the English nobility'. As war raged with Germany, to speak with a Teutonic tongue in 1940 in England was always going to be a tricky business. Predictably, soon afterwards, Trautner—this non-Jewish radical German dissident—was rounded up and incarcerated. Churchill, fearing the corrosive effect of so many free-ranging Germans in England, decided to rid his country of potential spies. These 'enemy aliens'—often a gross and unfair label—were to be exiled to foreign lands. And there was no country better to take them than Australia. After all, Australia was a place where the English had form when it came to dumping their unwanted.

To this end, Trautner was forcibly boarded onto the infamous *Dunera*. On the vessel were crammed over 2500 men of different political and ethnic persuasions—Nazi detestors and a few Nazi sympathisers—a hotchpotch of England's rejects; the vast majority were Jewish refugees who had fled fascism in Europe. Laden with this teeming glut of men, the *Dunera* departed England in July 1940 and made its way to Sydney, in much the same way as convict vessels did for the first half of the nineteenth century, voyaging and decanting its load on the Sydney docks. Trautner, at close to 50, would have been one of the older detainees to step upon the shores of Australia.

Trautner, along with his fellow travellers, was interned in the township of Hay on the south-western plains of New South Wales. From here Trautner was moved to Orange and finally to Tatura in central Victoria, 180 kilometres from Melbourne. That's when luck came waltzing his way.

Trautner may have rotted in an internment camp until the end of the war were it not for another remarkable man—'Pansy' Wright. Roy Douglas Wright was professor of physiology at the University of Melbourne, and had a 'habit of collecting strays' with scientific talent. A perpetual fighter for the underdog, Wright was made aware of Trautner's imprisonment and organised his transfer to the university to work under him in the physiology department. Wright turned heads wherever he went; he was coarse-tongued and swashbuckling, and had a large face whose porcine features earned him a role in a student review and the ironic nickname 'Pansy'. He was an academic doing all that apparently well-behaved professors were not supposed to do. For Trautner, the rough-edged 'Pansy' Wright was a godsend. Trautner's future was secured in 1944 by a man gruff in nature but abounding in human understanding.

It was while at the university that Trautner's roving eye settled upon John Cade's 1949 paper on lithium. Within weeks of reading it, it seems, Trautner had joined forces with a psychiatrist by the name of Charlie Noack from the Mont Park Mental Hospital and set about treating patients with lithium. With a stroke they had over a hundred patients on their books—the largest single collection of lithium patients anywhere—and published their findings in 1951 in *The Medical Journal of Australia*. John Cade had little to do with this paper; Traunter did communicate with John, but their relationship was a distant one.

It was at about this time that another man, eager to study lithium, arrived on John Cade's doorstep.

Sam Gershon, brash and breezy, descended on Melbourne in 1952 to take up a post as a young trainee psychiatrist at Royal Park. Born in Poland, and in his second year as a doctor, after graduating from the University of Sydney, he packed energy and enterprise in a featherweight's frame that peaked on a good day at 5 feet 4 inches. From the time of his arrival, Gershon sought out ways to involve himself in lithium research and to meet John Cade.

Gershon was precocious and smart; as a medical student, he had read John's article on lithium. Remarkably, even as a junior doctor in Sydney, he had had the enterprise to trial lithium on patients. He recalled this episode:

> my rotating residency included a period in the psychiatry unit at Prince Alfred Hospital ... The senior honorary was Dr George McGeorge ... he was in private forensic practice and he drove a Rolls-Royce and he was a very nice man and a very unusual fellow ... because when I discussed this [the use of lithium] with him, he said 'Look, we really don't know what we're doing ... we don't know what these diseases are. If this is reported and claimed to be something from this institution in Melbourne it's worth a trial. My only concern is safety.' I only used it in a few patients.

Infected with a desire to further study lithium, Sam Gershon landed on John's doorstep in Melbourne, one eye on ambition and the other on science: 'I was interested in lithium—why this particular substance had this extremely important, dramatic effect on psychotic patients.'

Although we don't have any written words to this effect from John Cade, there is a sense that he was, from the start, irritated by the youthful bustle of Gershon. On the one hand, Gershon was an outgoing, overtly ambitious man on the rise, and, on the other, John was a man of formality and reserve. It was a difference that never found resolution. Gershon's own reflections affirm this picture: 'We had a highly formal and slightly hostile relationship.' And as for lithium? Gershon's memory of his time at Royal Park is that John Cade had gone off the idea of lithium. He recalls that John 'didn't want anything to do with the use of lithium; he'd banned it, he didn't want to hear about it'.

Gershon, by the way, is not the only person who recalled John's reluctance to use lithium in the early 1950s. Dr Neil McConaghy, another junior doctor, who shared a house with Sam Gershon at Royal Park, had similar memories, and Pansy Wright, in a lecture at the University of Melbourne in the early 1980s, recalled that 'Cade had dropped lithium like a hot potato'.

So what was going on in John's mind? How worried was he about lithium in the early 1950s? Well, if you believe those who later sought to stake a claim in the history of lithium therapy, and who worked most closely with him at the time, very worried, perhaps terrified. John had sat before the coroner once; he was not prepared to do so again. But is this assessment fair? Or more importantly, accurate? Later on in life John never gave the impression of ever having lost interest or, indeed, faith in lithium as an effective treatment. And not everyone accepts the view that John dropped lithium at this time. His oldest son, Jack, retired professor of intensive care at Royal Melbourne Hospital, mused:

> This is misunderstood. In those days, in the late 1940s, when one published a paper, people didn't go on to keep publishing as they do now ... he was a busy clinician and administrator ... I don't think he felt the need to be at the front. He felt he had done what he could and left the rest to others with more research skills, to follow this up. He also moved on to other areas. He was always curious about what caused schizophrenia. He left lithium for a while looking for something similar in schizophrenia.

The most important voice in this whole debate is that of John Cade. But it is hard to fathom what John's thoughts were, and it remains one of the great imponderables in the lithium story. Curiously, John himself never reflected on this key period of uncertainty and, sadly, no writer or historian pressed him on the point later in his life. It seems though, that John's belief in lithium did, at the very least, waver. There can be little genuine doubt that John was troubled by lithium. The real question is did he lose faith in it altogether? The answer depends on whom you ask, and whom you believe. It is a flight of the biographer's vanity to think it is possible to reassemble the mind of a man from over 60 years ago.

Regardless of the reasoning behind John's willingness to let the use of lithium rise or fall during his early years at Royal Park, Sam Gershon and John Cade fell out before they fell in. So Sam Gershon, irrepressible as ever, looked to start his lithium research elsewhere. That's how he met Eduard Trautner.

Before arriving at Royal Park in early 1952, Sam Gershon, had read not only John Cade's 1949 paper but also Trautner and Noack's 1951 paper. From the start, Gershon was impressed by Trautner and struck up a close professional and personal relationship with the German refugee. There are many recollections of Trautner at this time, all memorable. This is one of the best, from Gershon's wife, Lisl:

> I knew him very well and my memories are vivid and positive.
> He was truly a bohemian. He was his own person; he didn't
> care about convention or what people thought of him. He was
> dedicated to his science, loyal to his friends, and he looked like
> Yoda from *Star Wars*.
>
> I've never seen anyone so wrinkled in my life but Trautie
> was unbelievably youthful. He chain-smoked. We all smoked.
> He smoked like a chimney. He smoked 'Players' ... He was
> a jovial person, jolly, a bon vivant. He knew things about art
> and music and Europe. Very European, cosmopolitan. He was
> devoted to science but he was also devoted to living.

Gershon's wife remembers these vintage times: 'we'd smoke, and drink Cointreau and Benedictine. We'd drink coffee and he [Trautner] and Sam talked a lot about lithium and art and Europe.' Then, with a shiver of distaste, she conjures a contrasting image of Melbourne at the time:

> Melbourne in the 1950s was very British, very white, very
> pink, very WASP, it was so boring. There was no good food,

so people like Trautie were unusual; the only restaurant worth
eating at was Florentino's, then Pellegrini's Brothers in, I think,
Bourke Street.

In a post-war Melbourne of comfy cardigans and trundling trams,
and where the average person's idea of nightlife was to huddle
about the radiogram on the mantelpiece for an episode of 'Blue
Hills', Eduard Trautner rose like a comet that lit up the Melbourne
skies.

Trautner's thick, heavily accented voice exposed with every
syllable his Germanic background, and in a country reeling with
post-war Teutonic sensitivities about 'the enemy', he made the
decision—like so many others—to do something about his telltale
name. He anglicised what he could; Eduard silently, by stealth,
became Edward. Even for an iconoclast, acceptance is important.

Trautner and Gershon—mentor and acolyte—laboured on lithium's mysteries during the 1950s. They were a productive team. As we
look back at them, they make an odd pairing: a non-Jewish German
radical and a Polish-born Jewish Australian. Modern Australia in a
snapshot.

While migrants were slowly remaking Australia's culinary
culture, they were also, it seems, silently helping to revolutionise its
medicine.

By the end of 1952 the newly anglicised Edward Trautner and the
effervescent Sam Gershon were experimenting with lithium in
various hospitals around Melbourne—but largely away from Royal
Park. By year's end, Gershon had left Royal Park and was working
at Ballarat Mental Hospital. Here he continued experimenting with
lithium. His memories of the asylum are unprepossessing.

> Ballarat was a hospital of near 1000 patients; there was one
> psychiatrist superintendent who spent all of his time locked
> in his office writing those long folio sheets of follow up notes;

I don't think he ever stepped out of his office. In addition to him on the staff there was one other resident doctor senior to me . . . and then there was me. That was the total [medical] staff.

[The hospital] was like a Gulag. You know, the 1950s in Ballarat, there was nothing there. A big mental hospital and there were the ruins of the gold mines; and a derelict city. There really wasn't much; I continued to drive down to Melbourne to go to the University. The work with lithium continued . . . I could do what I liked up there at Ballarat. I'd take the samples of blood for testing lithium levels down to Melbourne.

There was one day in particular that Sam Gershon should remember: 7 December 1952. On that single day, two patients died at the Ballarat Mental Hospital—Bessie Lorraine Hawksworth, a 33-year-old ex-hosiery employee, and Mary Vera Raselli, aged 41, whose sad and meagre life description in her file states simply 'home duties', though, locked in asylums, she had not done this for years. The coronial review found both patients perished from lithium toxicity; Sam Gershon was the doctor in both cases and presented his evidence before the coroner. Several months later, after Sam Gershon had left the hospital, a third patient died from lithium toxicity in Ballarat.

In recent years, when asked about his recollections of these deaths, Sam Gershon could not recall any details. In fact, he could not remember the deaths at all. But he did remember the general air of wariness, of nervousness around the use of lithium, which pervaded not only the mind of John Cade but also the minds of a string of coroners:

At the time there must have been a lot of deaths . . . deaths were reported in the newspapers that went to coroners' courts . . . I mean, a lot of them were reported by hearsay . . . and you can't really track them all down, like this bizarre one we heard but never verified that some farmer was using lithium citrate on a celery crop to treat rust . . . and the family ate the celery and some got lithium poisoning. Whether that was true or false I don't know but there were a lot of stories going around.

Back at Royal Park, John Cade would have known immediately about these further lithium deaths in Ballarat. He may have felt they justified his urgings for caution in the use of lithium; more likely this feeling would have been overtaken by his still strong desire that lithium might yet prove its worth.

As the year drew to a close, John may have spent time thinking about lithium and these further deaths, but it is unlikely he did so, for his world was overwhelmed by only one thought: that he might lose another child. John Cade had already borne witness to the death of his daughter, Mary; now his oldest child, Jack, lay critically ill in the Mercy Hospital in Melbourne. It would be fair to say that lithium was the furthest thing from John's mind at the end of 1952.

As John's children tell the story, Jack Cade—fourteen, then a student at Xavier College—had a life-threatening, but to this day mysterious illness. How his father responded tells us a lot about what offered John fortitude in life. David, then twelve years old, remembers visiting his brother in hospital:

Jack nearly died. He was at the Mercy Private Hospital for close to 3 months, if I remember well. He was ill a long time. I remember going in; he was wasting away. Formerly he was a tall athletic boy. Now he was lying in bed, his arms flexed at the elbow, skin and bone; and looked close to death.

John, of course, had no shortage of medical connections throughout the city of Melbourne, and he pressed the most skilled physicians to watch over his son. In particular he sought counsel and care from the man whom he regarded as the finest physician in Melbourne—Dr John Horan. But, despite lengthy observation and investigations, Dr Horan was unable to conjure a diagnosis, much less a cure. The family to this day believe that no precise diagnosis was ever unearthed.

Jean remembered this awful time:

> Jack had been desperately ill for 4–6 months . . . the nearest we could call it would be polio but it wasn't . . . he had pains in his legs . . . extraordinary pain and could not walk . . . His forehead, that was swollen. He couldn't hold things to feed himself . . . I had to lift him to the pan . . . his cry was 'Take me home, take me home' and the pathologist took blood every day . . . and he said he felt 'wicked pricking John's fingers' . . . when I put a bell by his side he couldn't press the bell . . . he said: 'I can't Mum, look at my fingers'. They were so thin there was no flesh on them.

Whatever the nature of Jack's illness, death was near. John and Jean visited daily, holding vigil by their son's bed, taking great store in the utterances of the nuns who nursed their boy. As David said:

> Mum and dad loved the nuns. The nuns offered them a Saint's relic, a little container with, I think, the bones of St Gemma; they hung them on the end of Jack's bed. I remember mum and dad coming home after visits to the hospital and both crying because Jack was almost dead. They were sure he was going to die.

St Gemma Galgani was not an idle choice. The Italian saint, blessed with mystical powers, was said to have recovered, miraculously (there is no other way for a saint) from a serious illness as a young woman. An outcast, Gemma Galgani was said to exhibit the religious stigmata of a dying Jesus, the *sine qua non* of transcendental experience. Observers swore that every Thursday seeping spots of blood appeared on Gemma's palms, and just as suddenly vanished.

Now, from what we know of John Cade, he kept very private many of his religious beliefs. He was certainly no evangelist, and he bashed no bibles. It is unclear whether he believed in a literal version of the Bible, but, whatever form his belief took, no one disputes that John was a deeply devout and disciplined Catholic. David recalled his father on one particular occasion returning home from the hospital, heavy-hearted—matters were precarious with Jack—and quoting the attending hospital priest. The priest had asked John to summon all his energies into one furious ball and to 'storm the gates of heaven' with prayer to save his oldest son.

And perhaps, in this case, prayer was all his son needed; not long afterwards, Jack, against all expectations, recovered.

Whether John really believed in the priest's exhortations, and that those heavenly gates truly buckled in response to tumultuous prayer, or whether he believed Jack responded to the medical marvel of a newly identified drug, cortisone—identified only two years earlier—John never revealed; nothing remains of his thoughts on this matter. But regardless of whether molecule or faith cured his son, John offered copious thanks to his Saviour each Sunday at church, attending with his customary regularity. And when all was done, John may not have cared whether it was faith or science that had triumphed. He would take his good fortune as he found it.

26

When the newly appointed head of the Mental Hygiene Authority—the debonair Dr Dax—cast an eye over the poor state of mental hospitals in Victoria, his first task had been to scrub them clean, literally. The hospitals were a sink-hole of filth. But an overhaul of mental health meant not only the scrubbing of floors, or the painting of wards, or the burning of urine-sodden bed linen—it also meant an infusion of crisp, modern ideas. To help this along, in 1954 Dax organised for John Cade to undertake a fully paid six-month study tour of the United Kingdom.

Jean recalled their astonishment:

> Dr Dax sent John, which astounded him. [Dax said] 'I've got permission for you to go to some of the places I was in, to find out what they do.' Dax had arranged all the hospitals. His ship was booked. And John said: 'I can't go without my wife' and Dax responded, 'you'll have to pay for her yourself.'

There was never a suggestion that John would voyage to England without Jean, so without seeking further financial support, he paid for Jean without protest. And the four children bunkered down in the psychiatrist superintendent's house, along with a live-in housekeeper.

This was no trivial jaunt to England; John had a first-class ticket and a fully paid extended period of study, enough in those more frugal times to attract some media notice. As reported in *The Argus*, under the headline 'Mental Expert for U.K.', 'Dr John Cade, medical superintendent of Royal Park Mental Hospital, will leave Melbourne in the *Stratheden* on January 19 on a six months' tour of British mental hospitals.' John was to report back, like a soldier on reconnaissance, and offer suggestions on how best to spend the 'half a million pound building project now underway at Royal Park'. Dr Dax would be waiting for him on his return.

———

John and Jean boarded the *Stratheden* on 19 January 1954, in Port Melbourne. The following morning John wrote his first lines to his four boys:

This house ain't safe—it rocks, like riding on an elephant.
It shudders and squeaks too and makes at odd times during
the night a sinister snickering—I think there are wallabies in the
walls of our room.

The last lines of this first letter—'John, David, Peter and Ricky— Jesus, Mary and Joseph watch over you, dear boys'—were to be repeated often on this voyage, indeed they were almost engraved on the pages he sent home. Then, not to let the ecclesiastical moment overrun the practical, he prods their memories with filial expectation: 'Hope you remembered dentist.'

John and Jean proved the most assiduous of letter writers, a craft so seemingly ancient in the 21st century that one can almost picture the Cades—quills in hand, blotting paper on standby—beside candle-light illumination in their cabin at night. They wrote two, sometimes three times a week; the letters reveal their deep affection for all four sons.

John wrote to his sons tenderly, yet with firmness. He chose his words precisely to achieve this effect. So, laced in among words of warmth are directions of duty and the importance of self-reliance.

John was careful to write his letters in sections for his boys according to their age—from sixteen-year-old Jack down to four-year-old Richard. To his older boys he would reserve the right for the odd blue joke, something John saw as a kind of ritual of upbringing for boys entering manhood. It is true that John was a devout Catholic but he was no puritan and he loved to stir the pot and indulge in a private risqué joke or two with the boys. Before he left for England, John's sometime saucy lines flowed freely when he spent time with his older boys, sprinkling his conversation with suggestive limericks. John had an encyclopedia's worth of suggestive rhymes, no doubt honed during his time in Changi, which he poured out at will.

> There once was a man from Leeds,
> Who swallowed a packet of seeds,
> And blades of grass
> Grew out of his arse,
> And on his balls grew weeds.

> There once was a woman called Rhoda,
> Who kept an immoral pagoda,
> And the walls of the halls
> Were lined with the balls
> Of the immoral young men who bestrode her.

Whenever one of the boys wrote to John with the merest suggestion of a sore throat, they received the full force of their father's considerable medical evaluation and strict recommendations of whom to consult. John was no hypochondriac but he still had his own worrying fevers from time to time, courtesy, most likely, of the endemic malaria from Changi, and his near-death from pneumonia while a young doctor. The sight of Jack lying at death's door was also fresh in John's mind. Penicillin had only been around for a handful of years, so a cough in any of his sons was met with concern.

Some fathers are cut off from their sons because of absence (long hours at work usually the culprit), some because of drink, some because they never connected. Whatever the cause, many fathers remain inaccessible to their sons, while sons, on the other hand, desperately want their fathers to listen. By dint of personality and time of birth and, perhaps, the dehumanising effect of war, John Cade's own father was difficult to approach. One can't help but think that John's stiff relationship with his own father, in which affectionate words were rarely uttered, shaped how he wrote to his four sons during this voyage. John made sure that lack of expressed love would never be the cause of disaffection within his own family.

The *Stratheden*'s first stop—Adelaide, in South Australia—allowed John to roam the Botanical Gardens, taking time to observe and attune himself to this green delight. He bent and studied lotuses with 'circular leaves about 2 feet diameter', measuring their delicate but expansive pink flowers as 'two hands breadths' across. And then as a small bird flashed past he turned and smiled, stopped and tried to make 'friends with a willy wagtail'. Wherever John roved he found a place for the patterns of nature in his roomy intellect. And while the Botanical Gardens was a favoured haunt in the natural world, the deck of the *Stratheden* was a habitat of sorts as well, with different species of passengers for John to categorise and make notes on.

Among the ships passengers, there were various notables and non-notables: both at different times intrigued John, who studied them in the same detached analytical way he might study an egret bathing in a shallow pool of water. One of the passengers John instantly recognised—Douglas Jardine, former English Test cricket captain, a supercilious man and superior in his bearing. John ran his eyes over the aquiline-nosed Jardine like a blind man reading Braille, to take his measure. All Australians knew Jardine from the infamous bodyline Test series of 1932–33—and they didn't like him. Jardine played the game of cricket with a ruthless lining that broke no rule but broke the spirit of the game; he was just the sort of Englishman to make John's skin crawl.

During the long days on board, John recorded that he observed an albatross 'skimming the waves', and how, on crossing the Tropic of Capricorn and entering iridescent warmer waters, schools of flying fish burst from the ocean in an orchestra of glittering salt-water spray. John carefully detailed how each individual fish gave 'a mighty wriggle with their tail fins' until it broke free of the ocean, using its pectoral fins to glide for a further 30 to 40 metres. 'Every so often one will let his tail fin hit the water and give an extra wriggle to gain a few more yards.' It was often the smallest of details that John troubled to record, as much for himself as for anyone else. Jean, in her later years, simply summed up her husband's life as 'one of observation'. Whether it was a pectoral fin, the flight of an alba-tross or the minds of men, all underwent the discipline of sustained studied observation by John Cade.

As evening fell, John brought his observational acumen into the *Stratheden*'s first-class dining room and studied his fellow passen-gers. And as he did so we get a bit more of a glimpse of the man—of what he liked and disliked. And what he most certainly loathed—show and pomposity: 'From the passenger list I see too we have a tame Marquis & Marchioness on board—I haven't patted them yet.' And in the British he found a number of 'snob-voices', also among some Australians, no doubt keen to be seen as more than colonial. He described them all—in his delicious vernacular Aussie style—as members of a self-styled elite, 'the snobocracy'.

> Mummy and I are collecting voices. Our favourite is 'snobjam', spread thick, either English or Australian.
> Bread and water for a week would do everybody good. Sleek, fat, lazy and smug—that's all of us—waited on hand and foot. I'm sure some of the snobocracy summon a steward to wipe their bottoms. At times I feel like slapping some haughty dame on her well rounded rump and yelling 'Hi ya, Mum—have yer done the old man's washing this morning?' Still, you

meet interesting people and nice people—hard working ones
who are having a well-deserved holiday . . .

And in case anyone wanted to know the kind of man that John
admired, it was the captain of the vessel, with a steady-as-she-goes
hand on the tiller: 'He is a quiet firm man who keeps good discipline and knows everything that goes on.' This was the type of man
John respected: undemonstrative and clear-sighted, uncomplicated
and honest. John, in his admiring portrait of the captain, might
well have been drawing a template of his own ideal of a medical
superintendent.

The voyage to England put John in unfamiliar territory. Without
the structure of work, he seems almost like a vessel adrift, becalmed;
hemmed in by an orgy of first-class excess and sloth, it was not long
before the constant consumption of food rendered him guilty of such
gluttony. He looked down and observed, to his dismay, an abdominal girth expanding in a manner that he could only have fantasised
about in his Changi days. Caged by the gratuitous opulence of ship
life, he hankered to do something real, with solid earthy objects:
a hammer with a few tacks and a shoe in need of repair would do;
maybe even his Winchester single shot to blast at something across
the bow.

Within the first few weeks of travel, John started to prowl the
decks, tracing and retracing his steps like a bored beast behind bars.

On arrival in England, John and Jean headed to the Ashdown
Park Hotel, Coulsdon, Surrey, their base for the next two months.
Appointments had been made in advance, so John's time was clogged
with hospital visits. For the most part Jean was his secretary, wife
and travel organiser, a triad of roles that weighed her down at times;
a mild resentment gnawed at her as the months mounted.

Not long after he stepped on to English soil, John received a
noteworthy letter from his father, writing from Melbourne: 'I am
sending portion of this week's *A.M.J.* [*The Medical Journal of*

Australia] in which there is an interesting article entitled—"Evaluation of lithium in treatment of psychotic excitement". The opening sentence began with a reference to the "work of Cade" in connection with this method of therapy.' If nothing else it, in passing, reveals his fatherly pride in his son's experimental lithium work. And it also tells us something about John; that it's likely he had kept up a keen interest in lithium. It is unlikely that his father would have taken the time to pass on this information if he thought his son had lost interest in this marvellous metal.

In Surrey, John headed to Netherne psychiatric hospital for a prolonged visit. This was Dr Dax's former hospital, the place where he helped pioneer psychosurgery in England. At the time, Netherne was a prestigious institution with nearly 2000 patients wandering its grounds. John was impressed by the hospital, particularly its printing press and, of all things, its sock-making machine, glowingly putting pen to paper: 'Netherne is a wonderful hospital. It has the reputation of being one of the best in the country and Dr Dax was largely responsible.' There was none of the hostility in John's tone that came to mark his relationship with Dax in later years. John was taken aback by the novelty of televisions, found even in the hospital: 'one . . . five feet by four feet in the main hall . . . many of the wards have smaller ones of their own'. Television would not arrive in Melbourne until the end of 1956. And with an exclamation of surprise, he wrote: 'They even breed their own rabbits.' Which, while presumably efficient and reliable in supplying a food source, strikes one as infinitely less interesting than John's own method of achieving the same end— wandering about the Bundoora paddocks with rifle cocked to knock off a bunny or two.

As the tour wore on, homesickness and cold bit John's antipodean sensibilities hard. At the start of March, snow fell in London, and for all its northern hemisphere beauty, John was aware of walking in an alien landscape. In this chilled climate, racing from hospital to hospital, John donned the same much-loved overcoat he had worn for eighteen years, with its 'frayed cuffs, button holes and pockets'. When Jean held it up before his eyes and demanded that he buy a new one, he retorted 'It shouldn't fall to pieces for another two years', believing that nothing should ever be tossed out. To keep domestic peace, he yielded to Jean, and graciously lost the argument. Within the family John would often proclaim that he only ever needed just one chair, indeed only one of just about anything. More than this was profligacy. He even took this to his love of golf; when playing the Royal Park golf course back in Melbourne, he'd happily chop around the course with just a 5-iron and putter, beating all comers.

From Netherne, John headed to the Maudsley Hospital in South London. The Maudsley, led by the Australian Aubrey Julian Lewis (later Sir), was England's premier academic psychiatric institution. John trekked in each day, catching a bus from Surrey into London. In between hospital visits he took the time to write to his third son, Peter, aged six, exhorting his young boy to stop writing with his left hand. Enticingly, he promised juicy presents on his return from England if Peter complied.

John and Jean crisscrossed England like any pair of travelling Australians taking in the sights. Dotted throughout the letters home are the picture postcard images we might expect—the House of Commons, the Royal Mews, Windsor Castle and The Strand. Jean blushed, excited and self-conscious, when she reported seeing the smiling bluff figure of Winston Churchill exiting 10 Downing Street, with a half-chewed cigar and giving his signature wave to a cheering throng of which she was one.

After months of travel and a crushing work schedule, Jean could see John was slowing down. Jean wrote that his body was wracked by high fever; John suspected malaria, his old nemesis from his Changi days. He diagnosed himself and quaffed quinine. Struggling on without improvement, the fevers came and went. His weight dwindled until, gaunt and lined, he was admitted to Redhill County Hospital, Surrey, in early May. The diagnosis, it turned out, was not malaria but viral pneumonia. After two weeks, still coughing but improving slowly, he was discharged from hospital, a weakened but recuperating patient.

For a spot of rejuvenation, at the end of May, John and Jean took the waters at Bath. The thermal springs, used by the Romans, had been rediscovered in the previous century delivering, John wrote, 'half a million gallons of mineral water each day … People have "taken the waters", internally and externally for years for a variety of complaints of which in the old days gluttony and gout were probably the commonest.' John was fully aware that some of the curative properties in mineral springs around the globe were attributed to dissolved lithium salts. If he did speculate on whether Bath's elixir contained lithium, he kept it to himself.

In his last days in London, John passed by the 'magnificent St Paul's' and travelled into 'the crowded and mutilated East End of London and into the drab countryside of the north bank of the Thames'. His words suggest travel weariness; sagging a little, he was more than ready to come home.

Jean was the ringmaster of this British tour—sorting out the quotidian tasks of where and when they should go, and what to see and whom to contact. As the tour drew on, her irritation with her workaholic husband wore her tolerance thin; though there is nothing to suggest that, apart from the odd exasperated remark, she was anything but a loving partner. She remained a compassionate and caring companion. The same could equally be said for John. Even during their moments of aggravation they were remarkably gentle with one another. One suspects most married couples would be happy to trade their own degree of aggravation for the Cades'.

27

When John returned to Melbourne, it was to his family that he first
turned his attention. Jack no longer hobbled when he walked and
continued to get stronger, lifting weights; he was now rowing at
Xavier. David excelled in Maths, boasting to his father of a recent
100 per cent mark in an exam. The two youngest boys played
around the grounds of Royal Park. Jean, for her part, immediately
re-established order on the domestic front. John's and Jean's exuberance at being home with their boys was dimmed by the death of
David Cade, John's father, just a month after their return.

When John returned to Royal Park hospital, he found it
was changing, and doing so fast. Out went the padded isolation
rooms. John called them the very essence of the 'awe and abhor-
rence' with which the public regarded mental hospitals. Down
came the dilapidated accommodation; up rose a new occupational
therapy centre, an entertainment centre and laboratories in which
to conduct research. Straitjackets were given short-shrift and
disappeared into museums. Dr Dax had set ambitious rebuilding
targets throughout the state of Victoria. Royal Park, the flagship
mental hospital of the state, was undergoing massive changes; the
vaunted half a million pounds of refurbishment was in full swing.
Everywhere at Royal Park one could hear the thud and clang of
machinery putting things together or pulling them apart. Almost

as soon as John returned from England, his relationship with Dr Dax soured.

As Dax recalled from this time:

> I have no doubt that [Cade] ran Royal Park in the same way that things were done in the Army. He'd come over at 8 am. I'm sure he expected everyone to stand to attention . . . Cade turned up at the right time. He was always at meetings. He had his notes and his reports . . . I'd put the buildings there and left him to manage them. I was overbearing perhaps; [Cade] had to fall in with it . . . Well, he was rather rigid . . . a person who had high standards and he was a very good Catholic and had high principles . . . he worked conscientiously around the day. He could always be relied on . . . he was a very good rigid administrator.

Several photos of John at this time—thin-lipped and dour—conceal his lively humour; perhaps this is all Dax saw. John's reserve confused some of the people he met, who came away finding him humourless; nothing could be further from the truth. If you listen carefully, there is a twinkle in almost everything John said and wrote. In the end it probably depended on whether John was among friends or foes; his admirers called him formal, his detractors rigid.

Dax found John to be very stiff, and years later recalled a difference of opinion about the new Royal Park staff cafeteria as evidence of John's neat institutionalised mind: 'in a typical John Cade way he got all the tables up in line in a rigid sort of way . . . I moved around about half a dozen tables [into a more relaxed format]. I turned round and saw him raising his eyes to the ceiling. I had no doubt he'd put them back by the next day . . . Of course, next time I went they were all in straight lines.'

Looking back, perhaps the tension between the two men was the inevitable heat of friction when two strong-minded men—both of whom had a deep love of the history and culture of psychiatry—collide.

It is hard to fully recreate the tensions between the pair but the undertow of censure is apparent in this letter from Dr Dax to John in 1955:

Dear Dr Cade,

Following the last superintendents' meeting I would like to stress the need for patients to be adequately occupied in a useful way. There seems to be a growing misconception that when people speak of social therapy this is a form of constant amusement for the patient which excuses them from following useful occupations in the hospital. Adequate occupation and a feeling of responsibility for the day-to-day work which is done in the hospital is in fact a part of social therapy. The privilege of attending the recreational activities and amusements should, subject to the superintendent's discretion, be dependent upon the patient doing an adequate amount of work in hospital . . . It is hoped that much more of the minor maintenance and side-works of the hospital will be done by using patient labour. There is much useful work that needs to be done in the removal of unwanted walls, the cartage of bricks to close ward gardens, and their cleaning and stacking . . .

And so this letter went on with Dax detailing how John should lift his game. Dax's grandiloquence was not to John's liking; over 60 years later, we can almost taste John's fury as he read this dressing down. When this letter was read out to John's widow in the year 2000, some 45 years after it was written, she remarked: 'That sounds like Dax . . . I can hear the uproar when that was read.'

John, for his part, had a rather broader idea of occupational therapy than Dax. He favoured the offbeat idea of giving the patients Australian Rules footballs to kick joyously around the hospital yards, without a neat stack of bricks in sight. Clearly John's notion of therapy was a little too libertine for his more authoritarian boss, and a disputatious cloud settled over the two men. It never lifted.

In the early 1950s, just before John travelled to England, a gentle wayfarer knocked on the Cade's front door at Royal Park. The young man, having noticed the unused loft above the Cade's garage, boldly asked whether they would consider turning it into an artist's studio. That's how Max Middleton, a young artist on the rise, came into the Cade family's life. Max, as it turned out, had just returned from a rambling painting expedition that had taken in Spain, Italy, Bali and half-a-dozen other countries. With characteristic generosity, John not only allowed this young painter, then just over 30, to use the loft, but also refused any payment. In return, Max taught John and Jean the rudiments of painting, a task accomplished with some skill by Jean and none by John.

With John's name increasingly in the media it was not, perhaps, unexpected when Max Middleton, a specialist in oils and still life, entered a portrait of John for the 1955 Archibald Art Prize—Australia's most-prestigious portrait competition—picking up a more-than-respectable finalist slot.

Throughout the 1950s, while John was preoccupied with clinical and administrative work at Royal Park, research on lithium continued in Melbourne. Edward Trautner and Sam Gershon had confirmed John's early work, that lithium curbed mania. But they also solved the huge problem that had stalled lithium's continued acceptance. The problem had always been this: how did a doctor know how much lithium to prescribe for a patient? The right dose in the right person cured mania, but too much and the patient sometimes died from toxicity. Trautner's work brilliantly solved this problem. Using a technique called flame spectrophotometry, they measured blood levels of lithium in patients. They carefully worked out what was a safe blood level and what was a worrying toxic range. Doctors could now give lithium with the assurance that by measuring the patient's lithium level they could avoid toxic doses. It was the vital breakthrough lithium needed.

Among the vast collections of the Museum of Victoria is a leather-bound prescription book from Royal Park for mid-1956 to late 1957. It shows beyond doubt that lithium was being prescribed, with eight different doctors writing 27 prescriptions for lithium carbonate over a six-month period. Lithium, it seems, was regaining favour under John's watch at Royal Park. With lithium more safely dispensed, the rollcall of the dead was over; the last recorded lithium death in Victoria during this early period was in 1953.

The enigmatic Trautner remained in Melbourne until the end of the decade, when, like some furtive bush marsupial, he slipped away into the night as mysteriously as he had arrived. He headed north to retirement and the amnesia of Queensland, a refugee again, of sorts. Colleagues fondly imagined him beachcombing on Heron Island, knee-deep in salty waves. When he left, he gave one of his colleagues a prized first-edition copy of Richard von Krafft-Ebing's classic on human sexuality—in German, of course.

The ambitious Sam Gershon, who had a close, almost filial relationship with Trautner, relinquished Australian citizenship and emigrated to the United States. He would have more to do with lithium there, and became its evangelist, preaching its virtues to the non-believers until the Americans eventually re-entered the fray— like their entry into both world wars—late.

28

John's reading habits were broad. He relished the works of Arthur Conan Doyle, who made just one visit to Australia, in 1920–21, recording his impressions of the Great South Land in his book *The Wanderings of a Spiritualist*. During that visit, one afternoon, early in October 1920, Conan Doyle, celebrated author and doctor, saw something he liked. He sat high up in the Members' Pavilion at the Melbourne Cricket Ground, closely watching a game of Australian Rules football. His gaze scanned the arena, then settled upon the players. He observed their athletic stride with a keen mind and sharp eye, like the most famous of all his creations—Sherlock Holmes. Conan Doyle loved sport, once describing it as the 'sometimes brutal, sometimes grotesque' activity that lay 'deeply in the springs of our nature'. And he loved the indigenous game of Australian football he watched that day in Melbourne, writing 'I have played both Rugby and Soccer, and I have seen the American game at its best, but I consider that the Victorian [Australian] system has some points which make it the best of all . . .'

It is quite possible that even as a youngster John Cade knew of Conan Doyle's visit to the MCG, for John read just about everything that Conan Doyle ever wrote; later John, unashamedly, replicated the methods of Sherlock Holmes in his daily psychiatric work.

Take for instance, 'The Adventures of the Solitary Cyclist', a classic Conan Doyle short story published in 1903. A Miss Violet Smith—modest, beautiful and accomplished—enters the famous rooms of 221B Baker Street late one evening to stand before Sherlock Holmes and Dr Watson. Holmes scrapes the laziest of eyes across her features. Dr Watson takes up the narrative and describes how Holmes picks apart his prospective client:

'At least it cannot be your health,' said he, as his keen eyes darted over her; 'so ardent a bicyclist must be full of energy.'

She glanced down in surprise at her own feet, and I observed the slight roughening of the side of the sole caused by the friction of the edge of the pedal.

'Yes, I bicycle a good deal, Mr. Holmes, and that has something to do with my visit to you to-day.'

My friend took the lady's ungloved hand and examined it with as close an attention and as little sentiment as a scientist would show to a specimen.

'You will excuse me, I am sure. It is my business,' said he, as he dropped it. 'I nearly fell into the error of supposing that you were typewriting. Of course, it is obvious that it is music. You observe the spatulate finger-end, Watson, which is common to both professions?' There is a spirituality about the face, however'—he gently turned it towards the light—'which the typewriter does not generate. This lady is a musician.'

As usual, Holmes was right on the money. Now listen to John Cade writing about how he observes a new patient as they walk into his office:

After the face, the hands reveal most. It would be true to say that at times it is possible to make a reasonably confident psychiatric diagnosis if one is permitted to inspect only the patient's hands. They reveal infallibly the state of tension. One only has to see the agitated crumpling of a handkerchief to realise how distressed a woman really is . . .

The cosmetic state of a woman's hands and finger nails gives many clues to her mental condition, her occupations and her preoccupations. It is even possible at times literally to measure how long she has been mentally disturbed. Consider the woman who has previously taken great pains to care for her nails. There is lacquer on each nail, but it is in bad state of repair. Quite a lot has rubbed off, but she has neither taken the care to renew it nor had the interest to remove it. Knowing the growth rate of nails (approximately 1 mm every ten days) and measuring the fresh unlacquered growth at the base of the nails, one finds, say, a growth of 4 mm, since the nails were last attended to. It is hardly hazarding a guess to infer that she has been distressed for about six weeks. Right-handedness or left-handedness is sometimes obvious from the different rates of wearing off of lacquer.

Ed Darby, a medical student in Melbourne in the 1960s, remembers John emphasising in lectures the necessity for scrupulous observation. Darby, though not a student of John's, made a special one-off pilgrimage to listen to the well-known psychiatrist:

I'd heard of Cade. I was a 5th year medical student. Cade was very keen on students and demonstrating things to students. That one day I went he talked about the importance of hands. How if you were a motor mechanic and had no grease on your hands you hadn't been working for a while. He was an astute observer. He then showed us a patient, a man who was sitting in a chair, not apparently doing very much, just making funny movements with his lips and mouth and was totally unresponsive. I answered that he might be catatonic and John Cade was a bit surprised. But that's what it was and he then picked up the chap's arm and it stayed suspended for some time. It made quite an impression on me.

John rather liked these dramatic flourishes when presenting patients to an audience. Sometimes it was a suspended arm, another time a wayward walk, and, at other times, it was a manic patient who proclaimed himself as the true medical superintendent of Royal Park and that Dr Cade was merely an imposter. But John was never careless in how he presented patients to his students, and was never anything but compassionate in the manner in which he interviewed them. He habitually warned medical students before his demonstration started to be respectful and 'never, ever laugh at the patients. But you may laugh with them.'

John Cade's lectures, held on Saturday mornings at Royal Park, were legendary among medical students. At 9 am, 60–70 medical students, like a flock of sheep, assembled outside and then filed in to sit, cramming next to one another, in the small tutorial room. There was a great buzz of anticipation, for the word had got around that these were the best lectures on offer.

His teaching was traditional, perhaps even old-fashioned. You rolled a patient out in front of your assembled students and took a history and tapped tendons, or in the case of psychiatry, asked more questions to reveal the mire of depression or exuberance of mania. And so the patients would enter, one at a time, and John would demonstrate, masterfully. He cast his eye over each component of the patient before him, totting up evidence for and against each possible diagnosis. In most cases he'd have this sorted before the patient opened his or her mouth.

One medical student remembers one patient, who'd grown a little stout, squeezing into a Richmond football jumper that had not been worn by the patient for nearly twenty years. There was a tell-tale scar poking above the jumper's neck line—a past suicide attempt—the story of which John gently fished out during the interview. Or there was the man who presented with the oddest of charcoal spots on his chest that confounded the assembled students. Guesses range from an exotic tropical skin disease to home-made tattoos. John revealed the patient was depressed and a smoker who habitually puffed away in bed. The patient was so depressed he barely felt the pain as the ash fell from his burning cigarette and ate into the flesh of his torso.

John observed every patient intently until he had drained dry everything that could be offered. The face told him most: 'Quite often one can make a spot diagnosis from an inspection of the patient's face; but, short of this, one invariably obtains vital clues . . .' He rattled off a list of what was front of mind when he greeted a new patient: who can forget 'the clicking mouth-moistener is usually anxious' or the 'frozen' face of depression. And then there was the 'hand-clasping entry of the manic, whose hoarse garrulity detected from afar announces the diagnosis even before he himself arrives to confirm it'. As an aside he noted 'invariably the insistent hand-shaker is manic'.

John detailed his observations with a brutal economy of syllables and was impatient with the wordiness of those about him. Taut lines connected cause and effect. Dr Dax once gently deprecated John: 'he taught things in black and white, the students liked that'. Well, black or white, the students devoured John's jokes and clever asides and his commitment to high standards. They cherished his Sherlockian deductions in deciphering the meaning of self-cutting on different parts of the body, and poured in through the doors on a Saturday morning to hear lectures they would remember for the rest of their professional lives.

Back in the hospital, John brought his theatrical bent to his daily rounds. On one occasion a group of junior doctors, waiting for John, noticed that he was peering out the window. Slowly they sauntered over, curious as to what was going on. John, now with his audience assembled, remarked: 'Do you see that tree over there?' Pointing to a tree in the courtyard he went on: 'I bet you in about 5 seconds a magpie will land on the grass under it.' The magpie duly arrived. Some of the doctors probably worked out that John had seen a magpie at the base of the tree tugging a worm, which it had dropped and flown away as John approached the window. John knew it must return for its fleshy food. Although generally an undemonstrative man, John was not beyond these touches of *coup de théâtre* to impress.

Puzzles were not just for medical students. John, playfully, inflicted them on anyone. If you spent time with John Cade you were bound to be put on the spot. All his four boys remember the dinner-time conundrums around the Cade table. It might start with John listening to questions the two older boys had from their university lectures that day—both Jack and David became medical students—and offering the soundest of responses. Then John would smile, lean back and launch into a puzzle or two. The boys recall:

> He had a couple of favourites. 'If a chook and a half lays an egg and a half in a day and a half, how many eggs does a chook lay in a day?' or on another day we'd get 'Brothers and sisters have I none but *that* man's father is my father's son. Who is that man?' But he'd never tell us the answer. You had to work that out.

John took great delight in pointing out things that the average person just blundered through, not observing. And it could be the weirdest of things, like his conversation one day with his youngest boy, Peter, as they strolled around the garden at Royal Park.

John abruptly turned around, faced his son, and interrogated: 'Do you know that an emperor gum caterpillar's arsehole is six-sided?' It was the sort of question to raise the interest of any boy. And any boy in Melbourne worth his salt knew exactly what emperor gum cater-pillars were. They were soft-bellied, thick-as-your-thumb, blue–green caterpillars that appeared each spring in Melbourne. The Royal Park property was full of them, a veritable army of marching caterpillars munching their way through kilos of eucalypt leaves, defoliating trees like a strip-mining operation. John pointed to some fresh leaves in the uppermost altitude in the eucalypts where the caterpillars were silently going about their work. In a flash John dropped to his hands and knees examining the grass. When he stood, his smile betrayed some mischief at work in his mind; he extended his hand towards his son.

Peter recalled: 'I saw these tiny six-sided pellets shaped like miniature hand-grenades in the hollow of his hand.' John proudly announced, 'Son, that's caterpillar poop. If you watch one of the caterpillars, they eat so much that you'll see a little turd coming out quite often.' His boy was more than impressed with the old man. Poop, in all shapes and sizes and from all species, was a continuing John Cade specialty, often to the social discomfort of his wife.

John, never shy of trying something new, had been inspired by the Italians living around him to have a shot at growing olive trees. And to his own eyes cultivation had gone well. Jean was less enamoured. Next came bottling the olives, as Jean recalled:

> I said, you don't know how to bottle olives. He said that doesn't matter I'll find out. So we had olives and you could see them from the back gate . . . We had all these Italians knocking on the backdoor: 'Could I have some olives, please' . . . so we said yes. One of the hospital staff was an Italian and he gave me a recipe for preserving and my husband did that and we had big pots in the pantry . . . John did it very well . . . John made some liquid stuff, vinegar and God knows what . . . we ate olives after that with the meals . . .

On one occasion John was stirred to do more for his Italian neighbours. Peter, his youngest, takes up the story:

> A lot of the migrants grew fruit, vegetables and grape vines in their front gardens, mostly over galvanised pipe structures. Back then, most Anglo-Saxon Australians couldn't relate to this practice and considered these structures unsightly for a front garden.
>
> From memory a migrant lady placed rat traps amongst her vines in an attempt to stop Indian mynas or starlings from eating her fruit. These are not native birds and are considered

a pest. When there was an article in the newspaper regarding this lady being summonsed to appear in the local court on something like cruelty charges . . . Dad felt it was unfair and contacted Frank Galbally to help the lady. At the time Frank Galbally was considered Australia's leading criminal barrister. It caused quite a stir when Frank appeared in the Brunswick court to defend the lady. My understanding is that he was successful . . . I don't know how Dad knew Frank but they appeared to have a lot in common. Both staunch Catholics, highly intelligent, always ready to defend the underdog and [both] Collingwood supporters. Frank was happy in the lime-light; Dad on the other hand would avoid the spotlight.

John was not content just to look out for his immigrant neigh-bours. He had increasingly turned his psychiatric attention to the travails of post-war immigrants. Take, for example, a headline article in *The Argus*. The journalist wrote of a young woman, just 27 years old, found dead in a vacant plot in Coburg, a working-class suburb of Melbourne not far from where John lived. Her frozen hand clutched a milk bottle; a couple of letters remained unopened. A forsaken woman, her suicide note read: 'I am just a sleepwalker, a lost soul in the universe.' It turned out that she had migrated from Latvia, a refugee like so many others, just after the war. The journalist sifted through her belongings and uncovered that she had recently been admitted to Royal Park Mental Hospital. He tracked down John Cade.

'We certainly get plenty of New Australians in here,' John said to the curious reporter, referring to Royal Park and employing the common phrase of the time to describe migrants. John rifled through the admission register and fished out the non-Anglo-Saxon-sounding names for the journalist. There seemed a disproportionate number of them.

John elaborated:

It does seem that the way these people are treated in Australia is a contributing factor in their breakdown. These paranoid patients tell me that they are being persecuted and talked about in a hostile way. The world is against them. Their hallucinations take the form of unsympathetic Australian voices hurling obscenities and abuse at them.

For the interviewing journalist, John drew an analogy with the POWs he cared for while in Changi and in the years afterwards. The migrant, for so long straining to find a foothold, often broke down mentally when some security had been achieved. In the same way, John reflected, that some POWs—who refused to buckle under Japanese oppression—broke down when they returned home.

———

John's post-war home life at Royal Park, like his mental state, was regulated and routine. After work, he continued his well-worn practice of raiding the home pantry and filling a glass with sherry, right to the very rim. It's the sort of thing you see in people who, having survived some form of deprivation, treasure every morsel of sustenance. And this pattern was not confined to home.

When John went out for dinner he never bothered with a menu. He knew exactly what he wanted. Best remembered are the times at the RACV Club in Queen Street. It was always a dozen oysters and a beer for the doctor. And before he ate the oysters, he counted them, and if short-changed he'd summon the waiter: 'Excuse me, I ordered a dozen oysters. I expect a dozen. Not eleven.' And, before the waiter's eyes, John, like a boy counting out his marbles on the playground, would precisely prise the oysters apart to count each and every one of them. It was a ritual that embarrassed his family no end. Mind you, there was never a hint of selfishness or belligerence in this, just simply that one got what one paid for. Everything had a value, and honesty, even in the smallest of things in life, was a moral to live by.

This was a remarkably settled period in John's temperate and middle-class life, with a stable ship to captain. In the evenings he watched his favourite TV shows—*Bilko* and *Hogan's Heroes*—and religiously listened to the ABC radio news, taking care to set his wristwatch to the pips of the 7 pm time signal. Then, politely excusing himself, John retired to his study and set about his journal reading, in the same methodical manner as the caterpillars outside munching their leaves. To the left of his ever-present armchair rested a pile of unread journals; to the right was the pile of journals just read.

Outside of home, John was still an accomplished ball player of just about any kind, playing golf and bringing home par scores at the local nine-hole Royal Park course with little more than two clubs in his slimmest of slim golf bags. At tennis, a game he still adored, he remained supreme within the family, whipping all the four boys at will.

On Saturdays he took his boys to the footy. Peter remembers going to Victoria Park to watch Collingwood. Victoria Park was the kind of place 'nice' people didn't attend—or if they did, they tended not to talk about it. The suburban footy ground was remembered best for beer and brawls, and that was just on the field. But, as Peter reminisces, it was in the crowd that things could get really sticky:

We'd be there, standing on the terraces, Dad and me, and the players would run out. It was pretty rough around there, and I couldn't see over everyone's heads. So Dad would find me a couple of beer cans and I'd stand on them for the duration of the match. The cans back then were tall and strong, made of steel. Depending on how Collingwood went the crowd could be in a good mood or foul. Dad used to embarrass me when he started supporting the umpires! I remember once—I thought we'd really end up in trouble this time—there was this huge cauliflower-eared Collingwood supporter standing near us and he started hurling abuse at the ump. Dad just as quickly started yelling support for the umpire. Everyone turned and looked at us, I thought Dad was a goner. As we made our way out of the ground, after the match, I told Dad to be careful around men like that; Dad just waved me away saying, 'The person you really need to worry about is the one who gave him those ears.'

On Saturday evenings, after the football, John and Jean headed into town with season tickets to the theatre, or took in the latest offering from the Melbourne Symphony Orchestra at the Town Hall, or went to a classical ballet performance. And it was well-known that—when the odd cocktail party for a visiting diplomat was held—John and Jean might be seen on the A-list of invitees, alongside various knights, consul-generals, men with a string of letters after their names longer than their own, and occasionally with Lady Bolte, wife of the Premier of Victoria, Henry Bolte.

Most middle-aged Melbourne psychiatrists kept bottles of red wine in a spare room; John Cade kept his .22 single shot Winchester rifle. And although he rejoiced in Tchaikovsky's *Nutcracker Suite* and hummed Chopin's *Les Sylphides*, nothing quite got John's blood running like a spot of pig shooting on the Murray River.

Peter, his son, takes up the thread:

Dad and I would often go camping up in the Riverina. I was about 14 to 16 years old. This was the early 60s. We'd go just outside Balranald, one of Dad's favourite places. We'd fish and shoot; there were heaps of wild pigs.

My dad loved it; he went walking, examining all the trees looking for seeds to identify them all . . . He'd know the prints of a sheep or a pig, then ask us questions about it . . . He was a good bushman . . . We went up at least once a year. We didn't have lengthy chats, except, perhaps, about football. He was a good shot; he still used a single shot .22 that he was given by his parents.

One of the things that fascinated Dad was Aboriginal culture; when we'd wander around Yanga Station especially around the banks of the Murrumbidgee, he'd come across one of the middens and sift through some of the shells and explain to me that this was an Aboriginal community . . . I remember once he started to make boomerangs and threw them. It was a fine art; he soon got good at it.

During the late 1950s and into the early 1960s John's fertile psychiatric mind was on the loose again. He wrote several letters and articles on widely divergent medical topics, liberating his discursive mind to take root in the most unlikely places. There was, for example, his letter to *The Medical Journal of Australia* on the perils of not drinking tea. John had this rather farfetched idea about the cause of 'Mongolism', which we now call Down syndrome. We now know that this is a genetic defect caused by an abnormality in chromosome 21, but this was unknown when John cast his speculative net. He had noticed, with his all-encompassing roving eye, that pregnant women often stopped drinking tea. Knowing that tea was high in the metal manganese, he wondered if just perhaps the cause of Down syndrome was a lack of manganese during foetal development. He shot off a letter to the journal. And what became of this idea? Nothing. It remained a dead stump, and went nowhere.

John then directed his elastic curiosity towards the cause of schizophrenia, a perennial interest of his. He again suspected a faulty diet was at work. He put forward the unusual idea that eating fruit, especially cherries, apricots and peaches, offered some kind of protection against developing schizophrenia.

Both John's stone fruit idea for schizophrenia and tea-drinking for Down syndrome came to naught. Barren ideas? Perhaps. When you present these ideas to modern academics the response is almost universal. There is a kind of embarrassed looking away, of polite disregard, or maybe even a fleeting smirk at the absurdity of it all. But to dismiss this work and imply that John Cade was naive (which is sometimes done) is to miss the point. This was the same broad-gauge idiosyncratic thinking that had led John to lithium.

If nothing else, John was prepared to be called wrong, even a clown. In one of his lectures to students, John reflected on the value of medical research and said one thing stood out to him. That too often medical research was conservative—that it played along lines that were unimaginative and did not strike out to pursue new ideas. This timidity, he went on, would never lead to great discoveries.

There can be little doubt that John was thinking of his own spasmodic endeavours as a researcher when he spoke those lines.

Although lithium had found a place in the treatment of the mentally ill, its niche was still small, and the frequency of its use desultory, even in Australia. In part this was because the United States had yet to legalise the use of lithium, and still feared its toxicity, therefore the marketplace was small; as well, other medications were discovered that threatened to usurp lithium. That they did not succeed in eclipsing lithium, which trundled along in quiet ambition, is testament to the fact that no other medication quite quelled the volatility of mood swings like lithium. Lithium was still used in different parts of Australia and in a handful of other countries for mania, but it needed a boost if it was to survive and prosper.

As it turned out, on the other side of the world, a Danish doctor—with a mentally-ill brother—was experimenting with lithium. It was this connection with the far side of the globe that would ensure John Cade's work with lithium was never forgotten.

29

In late 1963 John received a letter from Denmark. The letter was from a psychiatrist, Dr Mogens Schou, who, partly for personal reasons, had been drawn to John's work with lithium. Schou's brother suffered dreadfully from unstable moods and had been in and out of psychiatric asylums. Jean's memory of this early contact was clear: 'Mogens Schou wrote to John straight away . . . *I must let you know, my brother, was a patient in a mental hospital for years. I gave him the lithium straight away, and within a few weeks he was fine.*' And, while this intensely personal communication was pleasing to John, it was the subsequent Scandinavian work that proved to be truly phenomenal. One of Schou's colleagues, Poul Christian Baastrup, suspected there was something exceptional about lithium, something that had never crossed John's mind. The idea that Baastrup and Schou decided to investigate was this: what if you kept giving lithium to a patient after their manic-depressive episode was over? Kept giving it even when the person was well? When they did this they found something no one had anticipated: lithium halted future episodes of the illness. In other words patients were protected from getting further episodes of mania or depression as long as they stayed on lithium. Lithium stopped bipolar disorder in its tracks. The results were far from perfect, and it didn't work for everyone, but in a stroke, lithium's potential role in psychiatry expanded. Not only could lithium be given when someone was sick with mania, it could, like insulin for diabetes, be taken each day to ward off future episodes. This discovery would prove to be lithium's salvation.

Schou's work impressed John, and over the years their friendship deepened, riveted by a shared belief in lithium. Schou, for his part, pursued lithium with single-minded fidelity and, for the next 40 years, promoted its value in treating bipolar disorder around the world. Fortunately for us, some of John's early letters to Schou survive, and we can glimpse a relationship that blossomed to one of great warmth. The first of John's letters, penned in 1964, is a formal letter about chemicals and electrolytes, cold and technical. But this formality was soon to thaw, and the two men, thick over lithium and with a propinquity of spirit, came to delight one another.

Schou's correspondence rejuvenated John's passion for lithium. After nearly fifteen years of little experimental lithium activity, John's self-imposed mental embargo on lithium research lifted, and he looked upon this special metal with a refreshed curiosity. Smitten, John began to collect and catalogue journal articles on lithium, and we come across personal letters where his thoughts wander again and again into that area that so preoccupied him in the late 1940s. He annotates research papers on lithium; writes to doctors and scientists for clarification on the various finer points of their lithium research; and coaxes those around him to take up lithium work at Royal Park. John's resurgent interest in lithium saw him inspire the Serry brothers, a duo of brilliant GPs-cum-psychiatrists at Royal Park, to undertake research. Awakened from his hibernation, lithium was now all the go in John's mind.

It might seem odd to a modern reader that lithium—so clearly an effective treatment for manic depression—had struggled for legitimacy throughout much of the world during the 1950s and 1960s. There was the initial calamity of deaths from toxicity. But this had been solved in Melbourne by Edward Trautner and his team, by measuring blood levels of lithium. Toxicity was no longer a problem. So why hadn't lithium been fully accepted? The stumbling block, really, was the United States, which had not lifted its ban on lithium, imposed in 1949. Getting the United States to rescind this ban would be the critical step in lithium's acceptance worldwide. With the new Scandinavian research showing that lithium could also prevent episodes of mania and depression, lithium's moment of glory seemed assured. But lithium's acceptance around the world was never a fait accompli. And on the verge of what seemed like full acceptance, another hurdle arose and threatened to subvert lithium all over again.

In the late 1960s, a series of highly critical articles appeared in medical journals taking aim at the recent Scandinavian work on lithium. They expressed doubt that lithium could be used to prevent future episodes of mania and depression in bipolar disorder, and implied that doctors, in using lithium, were dabbling with something incredibly dangerous. These sallies threatened to scupper lithium's growing foothold in the treatment of bipolar disorder.

This time the criticism came not from the United States but from England, indeed from the well-respected Maudsley Hospital in London. The English critique was launched like a series of missiles. Indeed, Sir Aubrey Lewis, the Adelaide-educated head of the Maudsley, it was said, unflinchingly labelled lithium as 'dangerous nonsense'. So the tone was set.

The Maudsley critique rejected the Scandinavian evidence that lithium prevented future episodes of depression and mania in bipolar disorder. The authors of the articles on lithium regarded the promotion of lithium as a misplaced infatuation with an unproven and dangerous treatment. In one paper, it was implied that doctors who promoted lithium were the modern-day equivalent of those who once treated the mentally ill by blood-letting. Scientific civility, always a slender thread in the world of research, was now worn thin.

To understand where this criticism came from and how it was shaped, you have to first understand something of the Maudsley Hospital in the 1960s. Russell Meares, Emeritus Professor of Psychiatry at the University of Sydney, who trained at the Maudsley during the 1960s, has some distinct recollections:

> I went to the Maudsley in 1964 . . . and for the most part I enjoyed it. But it had a curious atmosphere; it was very, very critical; and they were very good at ripping people to shreds . . . they were very afraid of doing things that were psychologically minded because Aubrey Lewis, the head of the Maudsley, might ridicule them; so they didn't go near that sort of stuff . . .
>
> I remember the junior common room, and you were very much reminded of being the 'colonial' from Australia . . . I remember the fear of not sitting correctly, or of not speaking correctly. People were very careful not to say anything that could be criticised. There was a kind of game they played, of scoring points, an intellectual game. There was a lot of sparkling talent but it was a tightly controlled atmosphere. Aubrey Lewis, of course, was very clever. He'd start asking questions to expose the first deceit if you were presenting to him; it brought some trainees to tears. We were all lined up like ducklings: from Aubrey Lewis downwards. It was a strangled rigidity and the atmosphere could be one of cruel humiliation. Fortunately it never happened to me and I seemed to get on well with Aubrey Lewis, and, indeed, most people at the Maudsley.

The early Scandinavian studies did have some methodological weaknesses and, after all, nothing published as medical research should be beyond scrutiny. But the criticism from England went further than this.

Barry Blackwell, a young doctor at the time, was in the thick of things at the Maudsley. He is affectionately remembered by everyone who knew him as a likeable man with a warm handshake and convivial manner. He boxed in the army, and was once slated to take on Henry Cooper, who, of course, went on to challenge for the world heavyweight title. Fortunately Blackwell side-stepped this but was, in his pugilistic career, twice knocked out. His other pursuit was rugby and when he arrived as a medical student, 'had such bad cauliflower ears I couldn't get a stethoscope in them. A plastic surgeon operated on them . . . so I could hear with a stethoscope.' An impressive man with a broad range of interests, Blackwell recalls his early medical career vividly. Everyone liked and likes, it seems, Barry Blackwell.

Blackwell very openly admits that he didn't actually use lithium and observe its effect on patients; he and his colleagues were critiquing the methodology. But in the midst of all the verbal cleverness and the preoccupation with numbers, the most important thing got lost—the patients themselves. Blackwell is now happy to say: 'It turned out that we were wrong. Lithium was really the start of a revolution in psychiatry.'

Welsh-born Brian Davies, the first professor of psychiatry appointed at the University of Melbourne—a Maudsley trainee from the Aubrey Lewis era—summed it up pithily: 'I'll tell you, they [the Maudsley critics] never used it on a patient and followed through and saw the family. They didn't have any clinical experience with lithium. You only have to do it to one patient and family and it [bipolar disorder] stops. You don't need any bloody clinical trials.'

John Cade watched this all unfold during the late 1960s. To John it was all bluster and bulldust; he never had much time for British condescension. We imagine that he saw this as Changi all over again; the Brits wanted to take charge and bulldoze lithium. John simply ignored them and their criticisms. His son Jack, by then a doctor himself, recalls that his father was little affected by this debate: 'I think he was pretty set in the way he thought about lithium by that stage. He knew that it worked. He had his patients in front of him. That's what mattered. He was not the sort of man who let those kinds of harsh words from other psychiatrists ever bother him.' John just waited for it to end.

Further research vindicated lithium's role in preventing episodes of mania and depression in bipolar disorder. And when lithium's opponents were finally routed, John, with the killer instinct of a prize-fighter observing his opponent sink to his knees, wrote to his friend Mogens Schou in Denmark: 'K-Oed . . . in the final round! Your contention has been proven so convincingly that the whole world must be persuaded.'

And it was. The Food and Drug Administration (FDA) in the United States prepared to lift its twenty-year ban on lithium for use in mania. Lithium clinics, like fresh shoots in spring, germinated around the world. Research and publications on lithium rocketed—at last lithium had found its rightful and lasting place in treating bipolar disorder. Over twenty years had passed since John took those remarkable, almost unbelievable steps with guinea pigs near his home in Bundoora, and now the United States was finally listening to the evidence. With the United States moving towards widespread use of lithium, it was inevitable the world would follow.

There are many endearing memories about John's love for his patients. How he would brook no stupid administrative directives when it came to their care. If there was any doubt about John's affection for his patients, and his bulldoggish protection of them from mindless medical administrators, there is one letter about a Royal Park patient that dispels all doubt. It is a letter that makes you wish for a psychiatrist like John Cade on every street corner and, in all its fighting glory, reveals John's disdain for unthinking authority.

To the Public Trust Officer
Re: Doreen

I understand you would be happier if Doreen were to submit dockets documenting her various purchases. Forget it. There will be none forthcoming. Doreen's accountant is God. Unlike you and me, she has a hot line to Heaven which she uses very audibly many times a day and she has been advised from on high regarding accountability. True, at times she makes unnecessary, ill-chosen and expensive purchases. This however is an index of femininity rather than psychosis. She buys quite a lot of food too as her own purchases always taste better to her than the hospital menu and she has the appetite of an elephant.

She is also a chronic giver of cards—birthday cards, Christmas cards, Easter cards, new baby cards, wedding cards, engagement cards—to name a few of the occasions which she documents in this fashion.

This must run away with a good few dollars a year.

We do our collective best to see that she keeps her purchasing within reasonable bounds, especially in relation to clothing, but Doreen is an exceptional case and must be treated as an exception.

For example, she is the one patient in the hospital whom I have exempted from the annual chest X-ray survey for many years. No man is going to invade the privacy of her body. God will strike them dead if they attempt any such violation. This prediction is made with considerable vehemence and gesticulation.

In short, as I said at the start, you won't be getting any dockets.

J.F.J. Cade
Psychiatrist Superintendent, Royal Park Mental Hospital

The public trustee must have also considered John and his letter exceptional. And so, rather than anonymously file the letter into oblivion, he kept it, like a secret treasure. Years later the daughter of the Public Trust Officer dug it out from her father's belongings and (to the delight of the Cade family) returned it.

Of course, Doreen was held in special regard by the Cade family: she was their housekeeper and favoured companion. The Cade boys still recall her coming to the house, striding up the hill, in a 'Mother Hubbard dress and an apron' even on the most oppressive summer's day, donning a heavy overcoat and lugging a bulky suitcase to 'The doctor's place'. She always addressed John courteously as 'The Doctor' and Jean as 'The Missus'. She'd poke about in the scullery, polish the cutlery and take an interest in all the Cade brood's doings. She was exquisitely modest, refusing to disrobe for anyone. And in the bizarre way of the deluded, this prohibition included herself. For when Doreen bathed she did so in the dark. John knew his patients well, and he knew when and how to protect them.

During the late 1960s, John frequently travelled around rural Victoria, visiting country GPs and offering advice on care for their psychiatric patients. John loved these jaunts up-country; they were a liberating time to loosen the coat collar and sniff the air. His peregrinations took him to Ballarat, Echuca and to his old haunt of Beechworth. Best of all he loved staying in the old pubs and having a counter tea.

Often he'd take along a younger psychiatrist on these country sojourns—Russell Meares was one of them. Russell remembers John well from these trips, and, in particular, one memorable conversation they had over dinner in a pub:

> We travelled around Victoria quite a bit. We'd meet as much as possible in older hotels; it was something John really liked, the old hotels. He did like to see himself as a doctor, and, I think, he carried a stethoscope, which was pretty unusual for a psychiatrist. We did chat a bit about Changi, which, in a way, was unusual for war veterans because my experience was that they didn't talk about it. He talked about how they even contemplated cannibalism to survive. I'm not sure if the POWs

as a body contemplated it but it must have been he and several associates who wondered whether this was ethical or plausible to survive. It was a passing comment, just a few minutes; it was just a calling to mind something that occurred to him in Changi and he didn't linger over it. So in a sense it kind of fitted in with him being a very practical man and it also . . . . implied a moral dilemma.

Russell Meares was right. It *was* unusual for John to bring up Changi, on any occasion; Jean could barely wring a sentence out of him about the war. So what prompted this momentary rush of self-reflection on events 30 years earlier, we'll never know. And why on such a provocative topic as cannibalism, even if it was in the form of a moral dilemma? It might seem strange that a man could, matter-of-factly over a roast dinner, have a dead-eyed discussion on cannibalism, to reflect rationally on what he might have had to do to survive as a POW. But should anyone think John was a cold man, all it needed was just the right ingredients to reveal his deep humanity. And sometimes the right ingredients came at the most unexpected of times. Like the time he had to kill his dog.

For most of his life John had dogs, and held them in high affection. His favourite dogs were dachshunds. Several years before his chat about Changi in that Victorian pub, John's beloved dog Sossie, a light tan dachshund, nosed about the Royal Park backyard. In the disused stables Sossie found and chewed on a cardboard packet filled with green pellets—rat poison. Within minutes, Sossie staggered and fell, lime foam clogging his mouth. As the dying dog twisted on the ground, John ordered his wife and children into the house. With no antidote for strychnine, the lethal agent in rat poison, John calmly found his Winchester rifle and shot Sossie in the back of the head— then broke into inconsolable weeping.

By the end of the 1960s John was living a comfortable middle-class life. He had his family and his well-worn routine at the hospital and was respected within and outside psychiatry. Lithium was increasingly accepted around the world and was helping to revolutionise mental health care. John expected, indeed wanted, little else. That's when he received an invitation to meet the President of the United States.

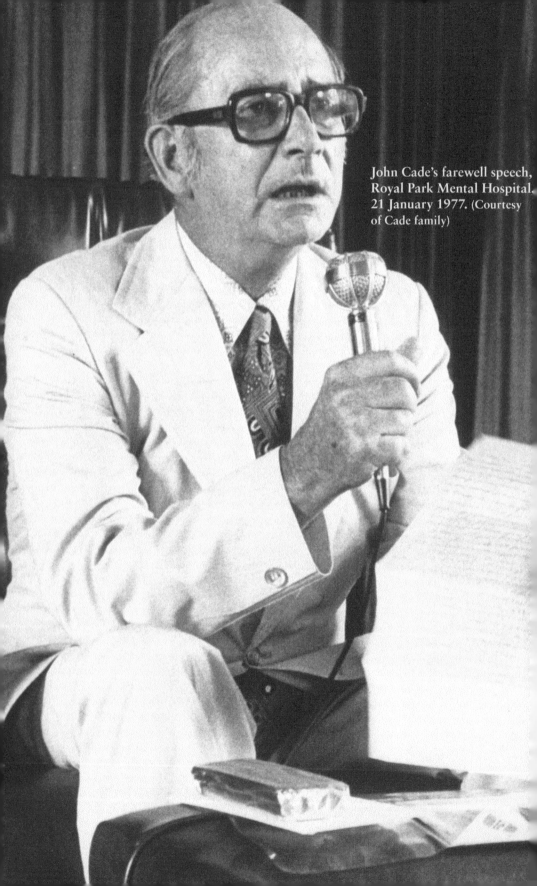

John Cade's farewell speech, Royal Park Mental Hospital, 21 January 1977. (Courtesy of Cade family)

PART 5

Even *the* dogs were barking lithium

LITHIUM: *Tales from a bipolar patient*

After a few months off lithium, I felt energetic, engaged, even electric ... I turned down jobs and burned all professional bridges with sharp and illogical emails ... I painted my face with spectacular green-and-gold eye shadow ... I stood on my head every morning; my apartment burned down; I served as the sole witness to a stranger's wedding on top of the World Trade Centre; I wore 800 necklaces ... I preached about Jesus wherever I went, which for a Jew is unusual ...

For two decades ... I have been taking lithium almost continuously. It has curbed my mania, my depression and, most significant, the wild delusional cycles that have taken me from obsessing over the value of zero to creating a hippie cult ... As long as I take those three pink lithium-carbonate capsules every day, I can function. If I don't, I will be riding on top of subway cars measuring speed and looking for light in elevated realms.

Jaime Lowe, 'I don't believe in God, but I believe in lithium',
The New York Times Magazine, *25 June 2015*

...e question of scrap iron for Japan, right any ho...
...was going to be done with it.

...that this Indonesian bid for independence is only...
...read dissatisfaction by the peoples of the East wi...
...ver lordship. The same problem is demanding solu...
Burma and Indo China...
...of political speculation. Regarding leave, idea...
...at 28 days immediately following disembar...
...k or so in a convalescent camp (probably at Bal...
...over-haul, followed by another 30 days leave...
...are not sure of yet is whether we will get i...
...cumulated recreation leave which would amou...
70-80 days. I suppose the department will...
...me as soon as possible — well, they will have...
...and I, darling, are entitled to a pretty good...
...that, I feel so rusty medically, that I simp...
...if possible three months post-graduate study...
...like to do a month at St Vincents, a month at...
...a fortnight at the Eye and Ear, leaving anot...
...swinging — all provided we can keep the depar...
...hen to work — as you guessed, in one of your ea...
...old brain box is simmering with ideas. I be...
...riod of waiting has allowed many of my no...
...try to crystallise, and I'm just bursting to p...
...test. If they work out, they would represent a q...
...the knowledge of...

30

On 4 July 1969, John Cade sat at his kitchen table having breakfast opposite his youngest son, Richard. An overseas letter, just arrived, lay unopened on the tablecloth—probably another enquiry about lithium. As John opened and read the letter, a deep smile split his face. Then, with the slightest of affectations, he nonchalantly turned to his son: 'I say, old boy, I've been invited to the States to receive an award and meet the President.'

Once the hullaballoo settled in the Cade household, it emerged that John had been awarded a prestigious medical prize—The Taylor Manor Hospital Psychiatric Award—for his 1949 lithium discovery. It was to be bestowed at a Baltimore symposium in April the following year, with President Richard Nixon in attendance. The meeting would be ground-breaking, bringing together for the first time in the history of medicine, the discoverers of major therapies within the discipline of psychiatry. More than a dozen eminent scientists and clinicians, including John, would have the opportunity of telling their stories of discovery in their own words. Travelling expenses would not be a problem; the Americans were footing the expensive bill with an around-the-world ticket. If there was a single moment when John Cade was catapulted from obscure doctor, who looked like a suburban bank manager, to worldwide medical fame, this was that moment.

Up until now, his family had known of John's work with lithium but perhaps not appreciated its full significance. That was to change after a deluge of phone calls and requests to speak to the media. Never ambitious for fame, John was, nonetheless, ripped out of his burrow like a bunny and into the glare of daylight. Discombobulated, he found himself in a celestial swirl of intense media fascination. And when John was elevated to the feature pages of *The Australian Women's Weekly*, he knew that he'd become, albeit reluctantly, the rock star of Australian medicine.

The reporter for the *Women's Weekly*, Roslyn Ross, visited John and Jean at their Park Street home, and immediately sensed that this was a man whose bearing and manner belonged to a different era. Slim in build, John moved and talked with due consideration, framed by an unassuming formality. Ross insightfully wrote 'there was something of the past about him. The "family doctor" of a century ago must surely have looked like Dr Cade. Tall and imposing in stature, with a friendly but distinguished face and a manner both gentle and sure, he looked out of time.' Those who regarded John as something of an anachronism in the changing world of psychiatry were now confronted with the reality that he was a spectacularly successful world figure. Because of him, patients with bipolar disorder were less likely to be hospitalised, and, if they were, recovery and discharge were earlier.

The *Women's Weekly* article exposed John and his work on lithium to the public in a manner that propelled him to centre stage, and he was asked to pontificate on all manner of issues. Encouraged to speak his mind about the future treatment of psychiatric illness, he boldly stated his views: 'We believe that many more mental conditions have physical or organic causes—not psychological ones—and therefore can be successfully treated with drugs.'

There was one oddity about this *Women's Weekly* article. When it came to how lithium was introduced, John related the story of Bill Brand; it was something he'd do hundreds of times in the future. The *Women's Weekly* stated that his first patient, Bill Brand, 'remained normal for the rest of his life'. This, of course, was not true. We all know that Bill suffered numerous relapses before dying from too much lithium. Perhaps this wasn't the place to tarnish an otherwise glowing story, or to detract from John's newly acquired American award. Or, perhaps, John was never asked what happened to Bill Brand, and the journalist simply glossed over his fate. We don't know. Maybe John felt that with the evidence now so over-whelmingly in favour of lithium it might do more harm than good to elaborate. So, as had happened before, and would do so in the future, the fate of John's first patient was never revealed in public interviews.

And as for Jean—after all this was to a readership of women—she appears in the photograph next to her husband, both of them bespectacled in thick dark-rimmed glasses. Her eyes are lit up, her smile spontaneous; John's smile is thin-lipped and calibrated. Jean is described as 'a petite woman with a bright personality' who it seems manages her husband's workaholic personality well. 'They are a perfect match. Even when Dr Cade looks serious she can make him laugh.'

When Jean was asked about their upcoming trip to the United States, she shrugged with more than a note of resignation and sighed:

> We might get a bit of rest and a holiday. Although somehow
> I doubt it. He is so involved in his work, but this makes me
> happy, too. The only thing that does scare me is that he persists
> in testing a drug on himself before giving it to his patients. I'm
> never sure just what is going to happen.

As the date for the Baltimore symposium neared, Apollo 13's mission—the third-planned moon landing—was spinning towards disaster. An explosion in a liquid oxygen tank saw power lost and temperature drop. The impotent spacecraft, like a crushed alumin-ium can, dangled in space. The world watched and wondered. Oxygen levels dropped; carbon dioxide levels rose. The rising tide of expired carbon dioxide in the malfunctioning lunar module was a chemical poison that would soon asphyxiate the astronauts. But the astronauts had one critical thing on their side: they had lithium. Canisters of lithium hydroxide rigged in a makeshift manner, and using some impromptu ingenuity, captured the rising carbon dioxide, converting it into non-toxic lithium carbonate. The astronauts could breathe freely again. As the astronauts scrambled to engineer a safe splashdown, President Nixon's eyes were deflected towards the three spacemen saved by lithium. The President sent his apologies to Baltimore: he would not make it to the symposium to meet John Cade.

Jean remembers the Baltimore occasion as lavish: 'It was all very extravagant . . . we were put up in a mansion.' The Cade family retain in their possession several glossy black and white photos of John's time in Baltimore. They offer a sense of the occasion in a series of snapshots. The first is a group photo of nineteen conservative-looking men, arranged in three rows like football players in a year book. John sits in the front row, unobtrusive, on the left, his signature thin lips unparted for the photographer.

The second photograph has John standing awkwardly in a crowd. Looking self-conscious, he slightly tilts at the waist, like a marionette, his elbows cocked at right angles; an ever-present thin cigarette protrudes from between his fingers. With his stereotypical thick-framed glasses, he is reminiscent of Brains in the TV program *Thunderbirds*. The final photograph shows John standing on the podium talking about lithium, peering straight ahead, above the listening audience, with a wide-eyed, mildly startled expression.

John's speech was characteristically gracious and modest. He spoke about his early days with lithium, his work to evaluate it, and his research on several other metallic solutions that might be expected to have pronounced effects on mental activity. Having been 'unexpectedly presented with a therapeutic magic wand', it was inevitable 'that one would plunge one's hand time and again into the same lucky dip'. The Baltimore *Evening Sun*, with a flourishing drum roll of American hyperbole (and with a misspelling or two), had earlier proclaimed 'the announcement of a new psychiatric drug will be made at the symposium by Dr John F.J. McCade, of Melbourne, the discoverer of the drug lithium'.

John did announce to the gathering that he'd been taste-testing another metal. He once quipped to a newspaper reporter that he'd eaten his way through half the Periodic Table. On this particular occasion, John had been swallowing strontium which, like lithium, is used in fireworks. The strontium solution had made him alarmingly ill. His son, David, remembers: 'Mum was so cross. We were, too. We didn't know what was wrong with him. He was terribly sick for a couple of weeks. He looked shocking. He was slate-grey in complexion.' None of this seemed to have bothered John, who noted some mild drowsiness and headaches but was otherwise well. He then gave this strontium solution to patients with depression and schizophrenia. The results, he suggested to his Baltimore audience, were worth pursuing.

Standing on the podium peering into the crowd must have seemed a long way from hovering over a sink injecting guinea pigs in the years after the war. As John delivered his speech, *Time* magazine, with an impeccable sense of occasion, announced that the FDA had finally approved lithium as a treatment for the manic phase of manic depression in the United States.

During the Baltimore trip Jean remembered hearing the occasional caustic comment about her husband's lithium discovery. The rumours suggested John's discovery of lithium was a fluke, and that his rising fame was merely the consequence of this extraordinary luck. Although John was a man not given to casual malice, he was rankled by the insinuation that it all came down to good fortune; it was a slur, unsoftened by time, that he would occasionally hear for the rest of his life.

Once the Baltimore speeches were over, elaborate plans were made for the formal dinner. And of the evening's event, the local Baltimore newspapers reported that 'The Most Rev. Luigi Raimondi', the Pope's delegate in the United States, would oversee the evening banquet at which John would receive his award. This must have been the sweetest of sounds to the ears of John Cade, the Catholic.

From the United States, John flew to Denmark. There for the first time he met Mogens Schou, who was doing so much to promote lithium around the world. When Schou, years later, recalled this visit it was not John's work or anything remotely medical he remembered. One impression in particular imposed itself on Schou's orderly Danish mind.

Schou took John and Jean to a medieval church, the 'Church of Our Lady' in Aarhus. The church is unusual, as it has a smaller ancient church hidden beneath the floor. Schou tells the story: 'The discovery excited John, and when the party was again up in the church he started to go over the floor, systematically stamping on each individual stone slab and listening. He wanted to see whether perhaps yet another crypt church could be hidden under the floor.' Jean remembers, from that day onward, whenever John entered a church in Denmark, he'd start hopping up and down, like a human pogo stick, crying out mid-hop: 'I'm just wondering if I can find another church underneath.' If anyone thought John odd—this balding Aussie psychiatrist leaping about Danish churches—we can imagine he would not have given a damn.

Soon after arriving back in Australia, John received a present from Mogens Schou. The Cade family oral history has about three or four different versions of what took place next but they all illustrate the same thing: John's love of a puzzle and the growing warmth between the two men. Of the various yarns the family spins, this is the one from Jean: the present was an amber pendant. As soon as Jean unwrapped the pendant, John, spotting it from the corner of his eye, jumped up from his own chair and rudely plucked it from her grasp. He took it away to the window and turned it over, carefully, in the light. After a moment's silence he exclaimed with satisfaction, 'I knew it! There's a small insect in it. He's sent us a fossil.' And indeed Schou had, a tiny fossilised fly trapped in the amber.

The pendant was a little experiment from Schou, who predicted that John would immediately look for a fossil in the amber—seeking the unexpected in the commonplace.

In the 1970s John's feet barely touched the ground as he buzzed about to all parts of the globe. At the start of the decade, he had assumed the position of President of the Australian and New Zealand College of Psychiatrists. Awards and honours piled thick: Distinguished Fellow of the American Psychiatric Association, Roche Travelling Fellowship through Southeast Asia, Chair of the Committee overseeing the first Pacific Psychiatric Conference; and elder statesman for this and that.

Now more than ever in the public eye, John could still come up with the unexpected. John was always politically conservative, and on religious matters his convictions, though private, ran deep. In 1973 he was asked to contribute to a medical symposium on the issue of homosexuality, which, at that time, was a criminal offence in Victoria. Psychiatrists at the time misguidedly treated homosexuality with electric shocks to dissuade patients of this sexual preference. John thought this intrusion into a person's sexuality by psychiatrists a nonsense, and said so. John comes across, in his writings, as the most compassionate of people and, as was his habit, he played down the role of psychiatry:

> I hasten to add that as a doctor I regard it as highly irrelevant and always mischievous to make moral judgments on patients' problems and attitudes . . .
>
> My own view is that a stable homosexual relationship is certainly not more psychiatrically abnormal than nail biting, or thumb sucking, or doodling or cigarette smoking. If homosexuality is perverse and an illness or abnormality surely deliberately inhaling large quantities of filthy disease producing smoke into one's lungs day after day should also be defined in similar terms.

Everyone knew that John was the heaviest of smokers. He was having a joke at his own expense.

> Anyhow neither I, nor any psychiatrist that I know, am burning with evangelical zeal to go out into the highways and by-ways searching for happy homosexuals to brain wash them into semi-impotent heterosexuality and so-called social conformity.

It took backbone for John to take this public position. The medical profession was far from a beacon of enlightenment on this issue and it was rare for homosexual doctors to come out and declare their sexuality; the hospital system of promotion was hardly sympathetic to their plight. But this was John's strength: his capacity to ruthlessly think through the issues and not bow to the politically expedient.

John increasingly involved himself in public health policy. And there was no more important issue than the problem of alcoholism. Alcohol, John claimed, was 'far and away the commonest single cause of admission of men to Royal Park'. Many alcoholics ate poorly, and so were vitamin deficient. This caused irreparable changes to their brain and behaviour. John, seizing the opportunity, introduced the policy of giving any alcoholic who entered Royal Park huge doses of the vitamin B1 (thiamine), in an effort to thwart brain damage. It was a brilliant manoeuvre and saved countless lives. There is no doubt that John's action was influenced by his observations of POWs in Changi, who presented with a similar picture of vitamin B deficiency due to appalling diets.

This vitamin work at Royal Park was almost as revolutionary as John's lithium research. It brought him immense satisfaction and it was little wonder that, in May 1972, he was called upon to give a public address on this matter for the Alcoholism Foundation of Victoria. That evening he sat beside Sir Edward 'Weary' Dunlop— fellow doctor, University of Melbourne alumnus, pugilist and Changi POW—a heroic figure from Australia's Second World War.

In May 1974 John travelled to Detroit, Michigan, for the 127th Annual Meeting of the American Psychiatric Association. Representing the Australian and New Zealand College of Psychiatrists, he was called upon to make a short speech to his American colleagues. Beforehand, in his hotel, John scribbled his speech on the hotel's notepaper kept on the bedside table in his room at the Sheraton-Cadillac Hotel. That notepaper—mottled and moulding—still exists, with the hotel name and address embossed at the top. It makes for intriguing reading.

Towards the end of his short speech, which otherwise was on psychiatry, John informed his American colleagues, apparelled in their suits and gowns, that he had observed the water level rising and falling in the toilet bowl in his hotel suite. This, he continued to the audience (which we imagine was now slightly uncertain as to where this was all going), told him that rain was due in Detroit. It is not recorded what his American audience made of John's discursive launch into the abstractions of toilet bowls and meteorology, or whether it rained that evening, but we imagine that they were left a little confused as to what this Australian psychiatrist exactly did during his working hours. Among John's possessions from this evening, there survives a program of the night's entertainment, suggesting that after his speech John and the aggregated delegates could look forward to the De Santis Singing Strings, and dance till dawn to the sounds of Bob Du Rant and his orchestra.

That same year, it was announced in Melbourne that John and Mogens Schou would share the world's richest prize in psychiatry—the Kittay Award. The prize was to be bestowed in New York City. In awarding this honour, the judges trumpeted 'lithium as the most important development on the frontiers of psychiatry in the last 20 years'.

Before John left Australia to collect the award, a journalist from *The Sun* newspaper tracked him down, finding him holed up like a brushtail possum at Royal Park in 'a rather Spartan little office, very Public Service décor, with green imitation leather chairs, drab carpets and grey metal filing cabinets'. John took the journalist through his now well-worn story of how he came across lithium after the Second World War. Diffident at first with his growing international profile, John had grown more comfortable with his celebrity and by now savoured every lick of it. As the interview came to a close, he picked up a white lithium tablet and held it before the photographer's camera, the circular pill nipped between thumb and index finger. John drew back from it and momentarily looked closer at this tiny pill, squinting, to study its mysteries all the more, and as much to himself as to his interviewer, he whispered in wonderment: 'The stuff is so cheap.'

And that was part of the problem: the cheapness of the stuff, as John so plainly put it. Lithium was cheap, dirt cheap. Most other medications in psychiatry, indeed the whole of medicine, were discovered and promoted with hefty pharmaceutical company support. A patent was then taken out, and, if all went well, millions of dollars were scooped up by investors. But not for plain old lithium; dug from the earth, no one owned the patent but God. Forged from the furnace of the universe, there was nothing new to patent. No man-made chemical trickery had created it. It therefore meant that no pharmaceutical company contorted itself to promote and push lithium hard in the marketplace.

Not that making big money was on John Cade's agenda. His son, Jack, remembers that when his father left Melbourne for the Big Apple to collect the world's richest psychiatry prize, John silently slipped onto the plane, carrying a lone briefcase. Packed inside was little other than a toothbrush and a clean shirt.

In January 1976 John Cade was honoured for his work on lithium with an Order of Australia, the newly minted awards that replaced the antiquated British Honours system. This honour did not surprise Ed Chiu, a medical colleague of John's at Royal Park in the late 1960s, and from 1972 to John's retirement in 1977: 'John Cade was the kind of person who loved his patients, lived with them. I learnt from John that patients are humans, never mind the diagnosis. When you grow up with them, as John did, patients are very much extended family.' And in John's world, that extended family included the carpenters, the secretaries, the cleaners, the plumbers and all the invisible hands behind the running of a hospital.

Ed Chiu fondly remembered, 'When I came to work at Royal Park, the first thing John Cade told me was that when you finish your clinical work, spend time with the artisan staff: the plumbers, the cleaners and the office workers because they know a lot more about what's going on around the hospital than doctors do. He often, in the mornings, had tea with them.' To this day, John's family believe it was an office worker, a pay clerk, or maybe a carpenter or cleaner at Royal Park Hospital who nominated John for the Order of Australia. Among these workers behind the scenes, John Cade was a legendary teller of stories and a keeper of the good. Whether or not one of these hospitals workers did forward his name for this honour we might never know, but it sounds just about right.

––––––––––

The letters John appreciated most, however, were not the frippery letters of honour that suffixed his name; the letters that mattered most were the ones from patients. Sometimes they were written by patients he'd cared for; at other times the letters that landed on his desk were from complete strangers. Soon after the announcement of his Order of Australia, a copy of an anonymous letter to *The Ararat Advertiser*, dropped onto John's desk at Royal Park. It was written by a woman, who gave only her first name, Claire. Claire asked, 'Why does it give me pleasure to read of the recognition in Australia of Dr Cade's work? A man I do not personally know?' The answer was, of course, lithium. It had transformed her life.

Claire was just one among thousands of women and men the world over grateful to John Cade. The image of John leaning back in his office chair and reading these letters is an appealing one. Perhaps this 1940s man, sitting at his government-issue desk, might have even allowed himself the briefest of self-congratulatory smiles—but whatever else coursed through his mind, John must have felt satisfied that his life's work was now complete.

31

In January 1977, John turned 65. For a man who oiled his life with a series of well-regulated rules, the age of 65 was the socially sanctioned time for John to retire. In 1977 there was no political pressure to extend one's working life; you were expected to graciously down tools, hang up your boots, clip on the pen lid—and slide silently from sight.

John did the rounds of farewell speeches and dinners and spoke intelligently, modestly, at them all. Nothing flashy about his attire—a loved cardigan or worn suit would usually do.

John said goodbye to Royal Park Mental Hospital on 21 January 1977, after a quarter of a century as superintendent. On that day, nurses, doctors, cleaners, carpenters and others gathered to hear him speak for the final time. The hospital's parting gift to him was a vinyl-covered Jason recliner rocking chair. There is an image of him—both comfortable and a bit crass in that 1970s way—captured by a photographer for *The Age*, in which John, wearing a pale suit, is perched on the shiny edge of his new gift, peering forward at his assembled guests. Dressed in the garish trademarks of that time—a psychedelic tie and flapping lapels—it all seems out of kilter with John, a man of a more conservative cut. In his hand he holds a microphone, like an Olympic torch, and before him, on the foot of the rocker, he spreads the notes of his farewell speech, as if he is back at home on the dining table. He spoke crisply, with not a suggestion of an 'um' or an 'ah' to foul his smooth delivery.

In classic Cade style, John challenged moral certainty and talked about a favourite patient, whom he called a colleague:

> My favorite prostitute colleague was 4ft 10 inches, seven stone and the terror of the Fitzroy Police when demon drink was upon her. Teeth, claws and stiletto heels could do terrible damage, and they did. But when the demon was exorcised, then she became the sweetest person one could remember.

He further extolled his 'colleague's' sharp sense of humour and said that, within the bounds of her own profession, she possessed the highest of ethical standards.

John and Jean packed up the bits and pieces of their lives at Royal Park, among which were John's Bible and bottled olives. They had lived virtually their entire married life within or near mental hospitals. Now they were to move to the old Cade family estate—at 655 Orrong Road, Toorak. It was a homecoming of sorts for John. As a medical student he'd boarded there with his aunt Rene, for a time. Eventually John and Jean came to occupy one half of this splendid mansion.

John continued some professional commitments, notably as a member of the Medical Board of Victoria. He also flirted with the idea of private practice—the prestigious 'Melbourne Clinic' tempted him. It seemed that Jean, after all these years, would get her way—a husband in private medical practice. But either the patients dried up, or John's lot had never been the world of the entrepreneurial doctor. He settled for seeing just an occasional patient if a special request was made. Almost relieved by the release from daily contact with patients, he set about observing the world from his Toorak home. Between reading fairy stories aloud to his grandchildren—*Rapunzel* was a favourite—John pottered around the garden, once finding an ancient-looking stone which he sent to the Museum of Natural History in Melbourne for analysis.

The Toorak home was an obvious yet odd choice: obvious because it was in the family and available; odd because John was not a man of ostentation and everyone knew Toorak was the city's most expensive postcode. John lived plainly, with the asceticism of a monk. Watching his pennies, he drove a 1973 Peugeot sedan, and to the continuing annoyance of his wife, he never threw anything away. So they lived a frugal life in Toorak, the swankiest suburb in Melbourne.

In February 1977, the University of Melbourne held a scientific meeting to honour John Cade's retirement. Mogens Schou flew out from Denmark and was an honoured guest speaker. When John was called on to speak he gave a talk as distinctive as himself. It had pretty much nothing to do with research, but he chaotically took a ride through medical history, like a Don Quixote of psychiatry, with personal reflections laced with humour. At one point he stopped abruptly and eyed his audience: 'I doubt whether any of you know what *Juglans regia* is, still less of its valuable properties.' This, part-question, part-accusation, came from nowhere. He informed his now-bewildered medical audience that it was the common walnut tree and quoted an 1883 source that the walnut tree's leaves were outstanding in treating certain forms of illness. And then, oblivious to his audience's bemusement and without skipping a beat, John returned to his lecture.

After the conference John took Mogens Schou to Healesville nature sanctuary, one of John's favourite haunts. Within minutes of arriving, John, without a word to his distinguished Danish guest, took off into the bush. Jean remembers:

> I had packed a picnic lunch and when I unpacked the sandwiches, John took his first sandwich and disappeared. Schou, looking around for John, said: 'Where has John gone to, Jean? I hope I haven't offended him.' I explained that he always did

that. John didn't spend time just gossiping. He was back soon with some orchids for Schou.

In July 1977, John and Jean were invited to the First British Lithium Symposium, where John was to give the opening address. This occasion was organised by Neil Johnson, a British psychologist who would later write the first history of the discovery of lithium as a treatment for bipolar disorder. Neil and John became the closest of friends. On the evening before the symposium, displaying warm hospitality to his Australian guests, Neil took John and Jean out for dinner. Neil recalls the events that night:

> On the evening before the Congress my wife and I took Jean and John Cade to dinner at a small country inn where, between the main course and the dessert, John presented us with a sizeable and clearly quite lethal boomerang, and proceeded to demonstrate the energetic arm movements involved in throwing it. Two elderly ladies at an adjoining table became visibly alarmed, and John's confident and loudly pronounced assertion that, had a kangaroo been situated at the other end of the dining room, he could quite easily have taken its head clean off with the boomerang, led to the immediate abandonment of their sherry trifle.

John had long been fascinated with boomerangs and had taken to constructing them with the carpenter's kit he had kept from boyhood. Indeed he became adept at throwing them. His son David remembers how at Royal Park Mental Hospital, an Aboriginal man, Jack, taught the boys and John the art of boomerang construction and throwing. Clearly, in England that evening, John was simply putting into effect the many hours of training he'd undertaken at Royal Park, and for which his English guests were quite unprepared.

When John returned to Melbourne he set about the task of writing a small book about the history of psychiatry—he called it *Mending the Mind*. Jean explains his ambition for the book:

> He didn't want it to be a technical treatise. He wanted it to be just something that somebody, anyone, could buy at the airport and shove in a pocket and if they left it behind it didn't matter. He wanted to tell people the simple things of his psychiatric life.

On the cover of this slender volume is a marvellous Bruce Petty cartoon—specially commissioned—showing a slightly maniacal psychiatrist lifting the top of the head of a patient to see what's inside. It is a book full of witty asides and intelligent observations. John's humour shines from page one, including one of his beloved subjects—the 'dangers of madness' from masturbation. Those who knew him well said that when John was amused, he chuckled and allowed himself an extravagant lift of an eyebrow. Eyebrows must have been buckling all over the place as he wrote.

In his book, John's language is, at times, blunt and flies from the page. This is John the boxer. He's not wordy, and there are no low blows, but, like a fighter, his words aim to hit their target with precision. Fearless with his medical colleagues, he never missed an opportunity to prick their conceits. Deliciously, he took aim at his fellow psychiatrists: 'this book . . . does not pretend to be a treatise on human wisdom, in which field the last significant advance, many would say, took place nearly 2000 years ago'. A reference to Christianity, of course. 'Quite bluntly, I do not think we as psychiatrists are any better at helping people solve purely human problems of the heart than man has ever been.' Professor Ed Chiu once remarked that: 'John has no fear of criticism; he is well established in his own self-esteem, who he is.'

John was unafraid of whose politics he might step upon—whether the left, or the right—or gender slants; it meant nothing to him if he couldn't square it with honest thought. In *Mending the Mind*, he pulled together what he saw as important mental health advances during his medical life. In a disarming act of modesty, in the chapter on lithium he made no reference to himself as the discoverer of its wondrous charms in taming manic depression. Such a refreshing lack of self-promotion seems unbelievable in our modern society, where every self-invested bit-player struts on the internet to the world.

John continued to receive letters from grateful patients and men and women he'd never seen: 'I started to get a lot of fan mail from all over the world . . . even the dogs were barking lithium.' One typical of many he received came in July of the first year of his retirement. It was written by a young man who suffered from schizoaffective illness, a disorder that hovers midway between bipolar disorder and schizophrenia:

> I write to you as a young man of 34 who was diagnosed as
> suffering from schizo-affective psychosis in 1972. In 1976,
> after all else failed, I was placed on Lithium Carbonate . . .
> I have made a dramatic and almost complete recovery.
>   I thank you from the bottom of my heart for your
> wonderful discovery of 1949. I am even hopeful of eventually
> resuming my life's work as a lecturer in German.

But not all 'fan mail' was well received by John. In late 1978 there dropped into his postbox a small parcel. It was a book on psychiatry, written by an overseas professor. The professor—who was unknown to John—went on to say that he was in the process of writing another two books, and he'd be thrilled if John would send him a couple of autographed photos so they could be included in these upcoming books. The professor, adducing for himself a close relationship with John, perhaps based on his academic title, finished his letter by gushing: 'Your discovery of lithium has opened a new era in psychiatry!!!' It was all just a bit over the top; John's instincts sniffed cheap flattery. For a man as formal as John, we know he would have bristled at the assumed intimacy when the professor called him by his Christian name. John was not a self-promoter and he cast a caustic eye over those who were. At the end of the professor's bit of bumf, John jotted with customary candour: 'I don't know this gentleman from a bump in the road— no reply. J.F.J.C.' These were gruff words but John Cade was not a man to stoke anyone's vanity. Ed Chiu remembered this dimension of John, 'he did not tolerate fools. If you're not genuine he wasn't interested in you.'

John's demeanour did not change in retirement. Never one to blaspheme—'damn' or 'blast' were the worst things you got—his temper was leashed at all times. In his second year of retirement he travelled to New York for the 1978 International Lithium Conference. There he met up with Neil Johnson from England, who noted that John was somehow different, 'quieter and more pensive', maybe even a little sad. Johnson went on that John Cade 'confided in me that he had quite simply lost touch with the majority of developments in the lithium field', especially the more esoteric experiments underway around the world.

Lithium had now entered the modern world of big pharmacy, where assembly-line drugs are constructed by committees, forged in factories and crystallised by computers. Lithium had been old-school, hand-crafted, but now it too had entered a different, corporate world. Lithium research was now an abstraction, carried out in distant places in multi-storey buildings. It left John cold. It was a long way from injecting the urine of patients into guinea pigs—an earthiness that John missed. Slowly he drifted away from reading about lithium and following the latest developments in psychiatry.

But, just once, nostalgically, he reflected on those early days:

> I returned from three and a half years as a prisoner of war of
> the Japanese mourning the wasted years and determined to
> pursue the ideas that had germinated in that interminable time.
> I was able to go my own way unhindered by advice, criticism or
> caution. This is important. I don't think it could happen these

days. One would be suffocated by hospital boards, research committees, ethical committees and heads of departments. Instead I was answerable only to my own conscience and personal drive.

Just about everyone remembers John Cade as a kind man. We find evidence of this wherever we look, sometimes tucked away in some corner of his clinical notes, just a word here or there of compassion. Although he'd stopped formally seeing patients, he was always approachable. Towards the end of researching this book, while visiting Beechworth, one of the authors met an elderly woman who'd grown up there; now retired, she had returned to see her childhood home. In 1979, she came across John Cade's name in a local newspaper and took the chance to write to him about her son, who suffered from schizophrenia. John wrote back to her, a letter she keeps to this day. This is a snippet of that letter:

> Many thanks for your recent kind letter. I am sad to learn that one of your children is so grievously afflicted. And God knows and you and I know that schizophrenia is a grievous affliction in spite of modern advances in treatment.

John then offered the kind hand of friendship and some professional advice: 'I would look forward to meeting you. I think the most mutually convenient venue would be the Melbourne Clinic . . . where I visit on Wednesday afternoons.' Even today, nearly 40 years later, memories of meeting John Cade bring an afterglow of warm reflections from this elderly woman: 'He was such a lovely man. He understood. I knew he couldn't really do anything more, but who knows. I came away feeling good.'

The war never went away for John Cade. He continued to meet his fellow POWs from the 2/9th Field Ambulance at their annual luncheons, events that brought back memories of the war. John, in turn, went back to Singapore numerous times, where he relived the years from 1941 to 1945. One of those occasions was always remembered by Jean:

> It was hot. He'd say: 'I'm alright I can sweat'. He just had his hat on his head and kept up the fluids. He was a tough sort. He said he had a good old greasy skin that sweated well. We did get to Changi gaol . . . We went to the cemetery. As soon as he got there he said he had to find John Park's grave. There was no one to ask. We had this enormous cemetery to look around. He said, 'You go this way I'll go that way.' And I kept looking to see wherever he was. We didn't know how long we'd be. Then, he held up his arm. By the time I got there tears were pouring down his face. He had found his beloved John Park.

Sometimes, John's written words suggest an unresolved bitterness towards the Japanese but those who knew him well would not agree. Ed Chiu, who worked with John Cade for over a decade, remembered this point: 'John doesn't show a great deal. But his Catholicism and Christianity underpinned a lot of his decision making. He would come back to these principles when he made difficult decisions. God created humans to be equal. Equality is a religious one not a political one. His forgiveness for the Japanese is very much a Christian way. He never joined the RSL; he never marched; he never bore grudges.'

It's true, John never joined the RSL, and he never marched on Anzac Day. Yet he met his men of the 2/9th Field Ambulance for their annual lunches with a certainty one could set a clock to. Among them he was still ribbed as the 'mad major'. John indulgently smiled and accepted this title; it was a typical Australian backhanded term of affection. There was no pulling of rank here; a sweeper of shit was respected as much as a doctor of men. That's the way it was; John was comfortable among these men of the 2/9th. No professional jealousy soured their conversations. John was among those he loved.

And so he found himself among them, again, on 17 February 1980.

At the head of one of the most beautiful boulevards in the world—St Kilda Road—stands the Melbourne Shrine of Remembrance. It's the war memorial that every schoolkid in the state gets to visit; you step up from the boulevard, up the smooth green slope of parkland, to a peak atop which stands the Shrine—a heavy grey pyramid with steps that sweep upwards to a colonnaded portico. Everybody in Melbourne just calls it that, the Shrine. On that February day, the celebrated elms sweeping down St Kilda Road were in full flight; an emerald foliage illuminated the city. John was at the Shrine, as were the men of the 2/9th Field Ambulance, assembled, respectfully, for that day was a day for memories. They stood on the stone steps and looked up towards John Cade. John was about to address them, and their wives and their children. He did so, we imagine, in the same clear way he spoke to his men in Changi nearly 40 years before, when repeating verbatim the BBC radio broadcasts—recitations that would have brought him death if uncovered, but that resurrected his men's spirits. This day the 'mad major' was back, speaking again. But this day was different. And John needed God's wisdom to lean on:

> My dear friends,
> This year is the fortieth of the comradeship that we have been privileged to share. It is a very precious bond that binds the living and the dead and today we pay special homage to those who have gone before us and whom all of us must follow in God's good time. We remember all those fine men who have died but particularly those whose memory lives on in our hearts.
> It is said that it is a holy and wholesome thought to pray for the dead. Why should it be wholesome? I have thought about that and I think I know part of the answer. We remember their virtues—their courage, their fortitude, their generosity, their wisdom, their loyalty: and remembering we

emulate; and are better people for it. One gallant comrade, and you all know who that was, was recommended for a posthumous VC which was never awarded. As we think of him and the brave men who died with him the flickering flame of our own courage burns just that much brighter and stronger. As we think of the wisdom and loyalty of our only commander . . .

'Our only commander'—that, of course, was John's God, to whom he'd been so faithful over the decades. And the 'one gallant comrade'? Well, that was naturally Dr John Park; his death on Singapore soil 38 years earlier was the deepest ache John bore from the war. If John Cade's spirits were still not at peace, and they weren't, then the good doctor never found a balm in life to soothe them.

Death would be the only salvation for John's troubled spirit. As he said to his men that day at the Shrine, death and peace would all come in 'God's good time'.

And for John, God was about to come a-knocking.

32

Among John Cade's surviving possessions there is a tiny treasure. It is a tan-coloured diary for the year 1980. In it Jean jots her memories of her husband's final year of life—his illness and, eventually, his death. One gets the impression that some, perhaps most of it, was actually written after John died, for the dates at times seem confused, as if she was reconstructing the events of the year. They offer a private glimpse into her world and, in the end, an insight into her husband. Each of her pencilled scrawls, usually just a line or two long, signpost the last months of John's life. Although we read of John's decline, it is Jean's emotions, rising and falling, that we feel.

Jean starts, seeming to know the outcome of the year already:

> How do I write about this terrible year, yet I must keep the dates, as I am so forgetful of dates—and these are so important to me. John said, '1980 is not my year.' How right he was and so very, very brave. So we start with Sunday March 23rd admittance to Eye and Ear Hospital for removal of cataract from left eye.

What presentiment of disaster he sensed we will never know. At least at the start all went well and the eye operation was a success. But soon afterwards John had a fever that drenched him wet and shook his bed. These violent rigors returned later in the week. Something unexplained was going on. On 30 March he was admitted to St Vincent's Private Hospital with a perforated appendix and remained in intensive care for two weeks. Jean, a nurse to the end, fondly inscribed in her diary 'such a good patient', from which we know John was not a man to complain. When his appendix was removed, unexpectedly a small tumour was found in his large bowel.

Just over two weeks later, half of his large bowel was removed. As John recuperated, his quirkiness came to the fore, even in the most dire of contexts. Jean wrote:

> Three days after having a bowel resection operation my dear John told his nurse that he had said this little ditty and 'it had worked'.

> *I sang a hymn to Cloacina,*
> *Soft but cohesive let my offerings flow,*
> *Not harshly swift or impudently slow.*

It is quite possible that John's nurse thought these lines the delirious drivel of a desperately ill man. It was, in fact, of all things a homage to Cloacina, the Roman goddess of sewers. For a man who observed and made jokes about animals and their various droppings, he couldn't resist, in his time of sickness, to concoct a ditty about his own. To the end he enjoyed a riddle, a joke, even in the face of cancer.

Jean optimistically charted his slow progression from bed to chair. She wrote of his discharge home: 'Now to get strong.'

While back in his Toorak home, news came through that the last of John's original ten manic patients, whom he had treated with lithium from 1948 on, had just died. John made a note that this final patient had been on lithium for over 30 years. When first seen, this patient had been wild and lusty, his inflamed words poured out undiluted, outrageous and sexual, manic gusts hitting hard. He bellowed continuously and strode about the grounds of Bundoora with the bravado of madness. He eventually recovered fully with lithium. According to his death certificate he held the most settled of occupations, a clerk, and, succumbed at the ripe age of 76 from natural causes—a heart attack.

At this point there is a long gap in Jean's diary, until we read the ominous words 'Now the terror starts.' In early September, John noticed some difficulties in swallowing. By the end of the week Jean scribbled 'Results bad', and we learn that John had been diagnosed with cancer of the oesophagus. The cancer was almost certainly a result of John's obsession with cigarette smoking, and although his sons had exhorted their father for decades to stop smoking, he never could resist fine Virginian tobacco. Further rounds of X-rays, biopsies and blood tests followed; on 16 September he was back home awaiting an operation on his oesophagus. He headed back to St Vincent's for his operation, due on the afternoon of 24 September. When his surgeon, Dr John Clarebrough, opened him up, John was riddled with cancer. The operation was cancelled.

Jean simply wrote: 'Findings—terrible.'

Oesophageal cancer was a death sentence in 1980; John knew it from the moment it was diagnosed. But his boys remember him being as selfless as ever, wanting to spare their mother and themselves. Even when experimental chemotherapy—primitive and brutal—poisoned his body, he never complained. The most anyone could extract from him was the fatalistic cricket phrase that was a marker of his generation's stoicism: 'Well, dears, I've had a good innings.' He dutifully attended all doctors' appointments; Jack, devotedly, drove him everywhere.

John rarely talked about his religious faith at this time, but those who knew him are convinced that it offered him the solace of certainty. In dying, his attendance at church never waned, attending every Sunday at St Peter's, Toorak. Undaunted by mortality, John set about the task of dying as he had lived: organised and not fussing, tidying up what needed tidying. With Christian self-examination he prepared to leave one life, and enter another. He called his son Jack over: 'Look when I go, I'd like you to organise the simplest pine

box . . . and I'd like to be buried in Yan Yean where my parents are.'
And then, closing his mind on that topic he ended with, 'Now, we've
discussed that. It's done', as if he'd just casually decided what he
might have for dinner that evening. And so with a clang of the lid,
discussion on death was over.

Enfeebled by chemotherapy, John sat in bed, unmoving, shoulders bent forward, his bony scaffold visible. He hadn't looked like
this since 1945. His mouth filled rapidly with stinging, bleeding
ulcers; swallowing was almost impossible, so Jean lovingly cradled
cups of water to his lips. John refused to be fussed over; Jean fussed
over him all the same.

On the afternoon of Saturday, 15 November, his son, Peter,
visited:

> We were sitting together on the verandah at Mum and Dad's
> Orrong Road home. It overlooked a lovely garden. I spotted a
> bird in the garden that I didn't recognise. I went inside to get
> Dad's bird field guide. It was a White-Plumed Honeyeater, rela-
> tively common in Melbourne gardens. I kneeled down beside
> Dad and showed him the picture in the guide. His response was
> 'Oh yes' and he said no more. I thought the response was out of
> character . . . I now realise how very sick he was when he was
> so uninterested that day.

The following day, as death tugged at John, and knowing his
fate, he asked his son Jack to drive him to St Vincent's Hospital.
Shortly afterwards, settled into bed in the hospital's intensive care
unit, John closed his eyes to rest. Jack left and John was alone.
Into the Melbourne evening John's dependable wristwatch marked
time, and for a man who had lived his life by the most exacting
of measures, he expected nothing less of himself now. Never late
for anything in his life, John Cade kept his rendezvous with death,
going out with the tide just before the appointed hour, a few minutes
before midnight.

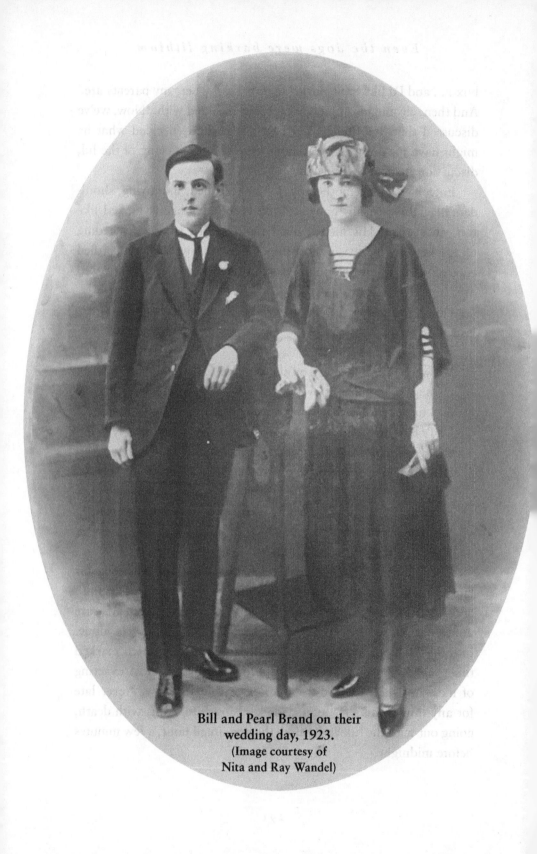

Bill and Pearl Brand on their
wedding day, 1923.
(Image courtesy of
Nita and Ray Wandel)

Epilogue

In the weeks and months after John's death, condolence letters poured in. Many now lie on Jean's old roll-top desk, yellowed and stale with the aroma of time. Some are from men and women with bipolar disorder; most of them had never met John Cade. People unknown to him mourned his death—patients whose lives were resurrected because of lithium. They wrote to offer thanks. This is one of them:

> Thirteen years ago, I suffered an illness which placed me in and out of . . . hospital for almost 6 years where, each time, I received ECT treatment . . . Each admission proved a longer stay due, no doubt, to my having developed suicidal tendencies when, on two occasions, I almost ended my life. I didn't want to live, but was petrified of dying. I had a loving husband and five beautiful, healthy children, but no feeling of love for anyone and nothing but hatred for myself . . . on my last admission, the psychiatrist felt I was manic-depressive and recommended I take lithium . . . I often wonder where I'd be but for lithium carbonate and continually give thanks to God for Dr Cade and his wonderful discovery.

Next to the pile of letters is an assortment of items from John's life—his dog tags from Changi, his well-worn rosary beads, his copy of the New Testament—spread out across the desk, entrails of a man's life. Lifting each item, turning them over, trying to fathom John's thoughts, inevitably there are questions. Some answers come from perusing his private letters; others come to us from the recollections of friends and family and (importantly) of those less well disposed towards him. All the letters—from friend or foe—point to a gentle, modest man.

Regardless of which letter or item is picked over and examined, thoughts and questions always return to the Bundoora Asylum in 1948, when John first used lithium, when he crossed the Rubicon and stirred a solution and handed it to his first patient, Bill Brand. Bill was always a bit of a mystery. No one really knew what he looked like; no photographs had ever been located. Indistinct and ghostly, he was defined by his medical records and the memories of John's two older boys. Finding a photograph of Bill, to give him an identity—denied him during much of his life—became somewhat of an obsession.

As the writing of this book came to a close, a photograph of Bill emerged. It came about by following the trail of Pearl Patten.

Pearl and Bill, we know, married in 1923; unable to tolerate Bill's illness, she left him. Pearl fled about as far away as she could from Melbourne without leaving the state, escaping to Underbool, a tiny town 470 kilometres northwest of Melbourne.

Underbool is a town in the Mallee district of Victoria, not too far from the South Australian border. Driving in to town you pass through vast wheat fields and plenty of red dirt and twisted eucalyptus scrub. There's not much to see in the way of buildings; there's a parched oval where the town's Aussie Rules team plays footy, although the local league folded in 2015—players were hard to come by. The 2006 Census recorded 217 inhabitants in Underbool.

Pearl lived in Underbool for the rest of her life. She first worked as a housemaid, eventually meeting a new man and starting a new family. When she died in 1994, well into her 90s, her small and exquisitely cared-for fibro and timber house—where she had lived her final years—remained untouched. Years afterwards, as her children prepared the house for sale, they rummaged through Pearl's belongings and came across a large, framed, oval photograph, in excellent condition, tucked away in her bedroom wardrobe. It was an unexpected find. The family had no idea of the photo's existence; it was a photo of Bill and Pearl on their wedding day in 1923.

When you examine Bill's face, it is not the smudged, damaged face one conjures up when reading his medical history. His face is like that of a Grade 2 schoolboy's: fresh, soft, as though his mother should be nearby to pack him off to school, or hold a hanky to his nose, or just be there for something, because you know that he will need it. Because he has the look of a boy, not of a man; his clothes are a smidgeon too big and slip skewiff from one of his shoulders. He has not worn these clothes before and he is unlikely to wear them again. It is a deceptive photo; he appears so uncorrupted by life, so unblemished, a sweet and beautiful boy. This is what Pearl saw before mental illness took Bill apart. It remains the only known photograph of Bill Brand.

No patient was more important to John Cade, or perhaps more vital to the history of psychiatry, than Bill Brand, the first patient treated with lithium. In the decades after lithium was found to work, out tumbled other medications to treat the mentally ill: antipsychotics to quell delusions and hallucinations; antidepressants for the morbidly depressed; anti-anxiety pills for the fearful. Modern pharmacies bulge with medicines for different mental illnesses—but the first medicine ever to specifically treat a mental illness was lithium.

If the story of lithium (and the countless lives it has saved) belongs to anyone, it perhaps belongs most of all to Bill and the other nine manic patients first offered treatment by John Cade. That's the way John may have wanted it, for John knew a doctor was nothing without his patients.

Lithium hasn't changed since 1948, nor has its value, though we still don't have a clear understanding of how it soothes the brain. Not every patient responds to it, and its dose still needs close monitoring. Although lithium itself hasn't changed, the way we understand bipolar disorder has. When John experimented with lithium, manic depression, as he knew it, was a uniformly appalling condition in which sufferers might remain in hospital for weeks, months and sometimes years. Over the 70 years since John started his experiments, the concept of bipolar disorder has expanded. We now include many milder cases where the highs and lows are not as devastating. Lithium remains at its most effective for severe cases of bipolar disorder.

John Cade—a true blue-blood of world medicine—occupies a rare perch. By showing that a simple chemical could help tame bipolar disorder, in a stroke, he turned our understanding of mental illness on its head. John's enduring legacy, lithium—a chemical born at the start of the universe—is found all around us, in the crust of the earth upon which we live. His discovery of lithium treatment stands as a matchless accomplishment in the history of Australian psychiatry, an imperishable moment in medical history.

When lithium was first stirred by John Cade, alone in the backroom of a mental hospital, in circumstances barely credible, a revolution in the care of the mentally ill flickered into life. At last we had something that worked, something almost beyond belief: a simple salt of the earth that was a balm for a troubled spirit.

Acknowledgements

My interest in the John Cade story was first aroused while a medical student at the Royal Melbourne Hospital. As a fifth-year student, and lost for something to do, I sat down in the hospital library and read through Dr Cade's slim but remarkable book, *Mending the Mind*. It was a moment I have never forgotten. In 2010 I was fortunate to meet Ann Westmore, who had completed an exceptional PhD looking at aspects of the John Cade story. From that point on we resolved to continue the research and complete a biography.

The interest and energies of so many in the Cade family over many years allowed much material to be recorded and used. Warm invitations were received from all the four Cade boys and I spent considerable time chatting and recording their memories over coffee and perusing the extensive collection of memorabilia and letters they had kept.

Jack Cade was always welcoming, urbane and charming. His stupendous memory, like that of his brother David, was a storehouse for a biographer. David Cade wrote some superb memories of his father, and they were of a great assistance in drawing out the life of his father. Likewise, the two younger sons, Peter and Richard Cade, were unstintingly helpful. Peter's daughters—Mindy and Anita—were also most hospitable, offering childhood recollections of their grandfather.

Locating the Wandel family, with their memories and memorabilia, was a wonderful moment and filled numerous gaps in the story.

The bibliography in this book includes a list of people we interviewed at different times over a span of nearly twenty years. To everyone we spoke to, your memories were crucial in piecing together this wonderful Australian story. Of this interview list, we would particularly like to mention Professor Barry Blackwell and Professor Sam Gershon; both live overseas, and took the time to speak openly and honestly about their experiences. Both are impressive individuals and we are deeply indebted to them.

We also had the good fortune to hear the memories of Professor Russell Meares and the recollections of his father, Ainslie, which took us back to the key period of the 1950s and 1960s.

Doug Craig, a former administrator at Beechworth, kindly took me on tours about the old Beechworth Asylum, and his wife, Val, was most hospitable during my stay.

Professional genealogist Peter Gill, as on many occasions before for my research, sourced many important documents. This would not be the book it is without his expertise.

In terms of written material, there was much to examine. Some of this we have outlined in the bibliography. Mention must be made of Professor Johan Schioldann's masterly work on the history of lithium—a must-read for any student in this area.

We would like to thank the staff at Allen & Unwin, especially Sue Hines, Angela Handley and Patrick Gallagher, who have supported this book from the start.

Staff at so many institutions assisted—National Archives of Australia, Australian War Memorial, Royal Melbourne Hospital Library, Brownless Medical Library, the State Library of NSW, the State Library of Victoria, State Records at Kingswood, NSW, and the archival services at Scotch College, Melbourne. Of special mention, I'd like to record the contributions of Tracy McDonald, Sandra Dayao at the Cumberland Hospital library, and all the staff in Medical Records at Cumberland Hospital.

Acknowledgements

Finally, to the following individuals who, while not included in the bibliography of sources, all contributed to the final outcome of this book: Tricia Atkin, Enda Bannan, Phil Boyce, Bruce Brand, Sheila Bruhn, Carolan Dodd, Di Elliott, Val Gregory, Shirley Mewett, Leoné Morgan, Maurice Sainsbury and Nigel Starck.

Taking time off from my medical work to write the manuscript required the support of the Westmead hospital administration and in particular I thank Dr Peter Cohen and Professor John Wheatley for agreeing to my leave request.

And finally to Laraine Emberson in New York City for her last minute 'run-around', a big thank-you.

Greg de Moore

This book had its beginnings at the University of Melbourne during my PhD thesis. A great debt is owed to the university for providing crucial financial and institutional support to enable the research that was the genesis of this book, and to my mentors, Dr Warwick Anderson and Dr Janet McCalman, who assisted my incursions into the world of the history of Australian psychiatry. It was at this time, in the process of exploring contested explanations for serious mental illnesses, that members of the Cade family and many former mental health professionals initially gave generously of their recollections, time and memorabilia.

Later, after Greg and I had resolved to pursue this joint biographical project, we were assisted further by members of the Cade family and many others, who provided a rich variety of observation and insight, greatly enhancing our efforts to capture the spirit, flavour and character of John Cade. We were helped along the way by many knowledgeable archivists and librarians who contributed their time and expertise, in particular Cassie May and Claire Watson at the Bundoora Homestead, Jacky Healy at the University of Melbourne Medical History Museum, and the staff of the Public Record Office of Victoria, the Wellcome Institute Library in London, the Australian War Memorial, the UK National Archives and the London School of Hygiene and Tropical Medicine.

Ann Westmore

Authors' note

The language adopted in this biography includes much that was commonplace during the period in question. Some of this, we would now consider crude and derogatory—especially as it pertains to patients in mental hospitals or some of the descriptions from Changi during the Second World War. Nonetheless, to maintain any degree of authenticity, the language of the day, particularly in quotations, was vital to the authors in recreating the atmosphere of the times.

We would like to note that, for the most part, we have been true to the names of all individuals mentioned in this book. Names of patients have been preserved, though in many cases we only had access to first names or surnames. Details of patients are in most instances readily available on the public record. Both authors feel that during long periods of incarceration many patients—through institutionalisation—were stripped of their identities. To continue this practice of denying them an identity, so many years after the events that this book describes, we feel would be a further insult. So we have, wherever possible, included the names of all concerned.

We would also like to acknowledge that the quote from Winston Churchill was first accessed in the book *A War of Nerves*, and that the quotation from Private Nicholson was accessed from the book *Carrying On*.

Select bibliography

Archival sources

Australian War Memorial service records of William Brand and John Cade, and Repatriation Commission Records from 1916, NAA, B73, M37180

London School of Hygiene and Tropical Medicine, GB 0809 Nutrition files

Museum of Victoria, Royal Park Mental Hospital Prescription Book, 1 June 1956 to 18 September 1957, Victorian Psychiatric Services Collection, Reg. no. 85.90

Public Record Office of Victoria (PROV) Coroner's Inquests 1950/25; 1950/1485; 1952/941; 1952/1866; 1952/1884; 1953/925

PROV, VPRS 6345/P0/367 (647) Bundoora Repatriation Mental Hospital General Correspondence File (1956–1981)

PROV, VPRS 6345/P0/245 Mental Health—Conditions of Staff in Mental Hospitals (December 1944–November 1967)

PROV, VPRS 2385/2 Parcel 23 Dangerous Drugs—Control of Mental Hospitals 1953–54, letters re dispensing of medicines in Metropolitan Mental Hospitals dated 10 November 1953 and 7 December 1953

UK National Archives PIN 15/28921 Conditions at Changi 1942–43; PIN 15/3539 Historical Notes by R. Powell, 28 May 1946

University of Melbourne Medical History Museum, Cade, J.F.J.'s
 patient history and reference cards related to therapeutic
 lithium research undertaken at Bundoora Repatriation Mental
 Hospital in the late 1940s, donated by Mrs Jean Cade
WA Register of Deaths for 1950, no. 84

Extended conversations with the author(s)
Dr Richard and Peney Cade, Fr Maurice Catarinich, Barbara
Cytowicz, Dr Elizabeth Dax AM, Susannah Dax, Dr Madonna
Grehan, Gabrielle Haveaux, Professor Frank Hird, Elizabeth Pren-
dergast, Dr Frank Prendergast Jnr, Margaret Rush, Thea Rush (née
Catarinich), Dr Susan Sherson, Dr Terry Smith, Joanne Wandel and
Mr David Weatherill

Recorded interviews
Shirley Andrews, 25 November 1999
Professor Barry Blackwell, 22 May 2015
Mabel Body, 25 August 2010
Jean Cade, numerous interviews, 2 December 1998–24 December
 2000
Dr John ('Jack') Cade, numerous interviews, 17 February 1999–
 28 March 2012
Dr David Cade, numerous interviews, 14 December 2010–30
 March 2011
Peter Cade, 25 August 2010
Dr Lloyd Cahill, 23 September 2010
Professor Ed Chiu, 30 March 2005 and 20 April 2011
Doug and Val Craig, 9 July 2013
Dr Eric Cunningham Dax, numerous interviews, 5 July 1997–
 3 November 2005
Dr Ed Darby, 20 September 2013
Professor Brian Davies, 5 April 2011
Dr Graham Edwards, 9 August 2011
David Elder, 23 September 1999
W.A. ('Bill') Flowers, 18 February 1999 and 24 August 2010

Lisl Gershon, 2 November 2010
Professor Sam Gershon, numerous interviews, 20 October 2010–
    22 December 2012
Professor Gordon Johnson, 24 August 2010
Dr Jerzy Krupinski, 16 November 1998
Ray Marginson, 19 January 2011
Professor Russell Meares, 9 August 2011
Dr Pat Melia, 17 September 2010
Dr Michael and Judy Messer, 11 November 2011
Dr Frank Prendergast Snr, December 1999
Bill Schmitt, 13 October 2010
Dr Alan Stoller, 12 November 1998 and 18 November 1998
Nita and Ray Wandel, 10 June 2015

Audiovisual sources
'Hindsight', ABC Radio, Interview with Stan Alchin, 'Behind the
    Ha-Ha Walls', November 2001
Troubled Minds, SBS Television documentary on John Cade and
    the discovery of lithium, 2004

Published texts, newspaper and journal articles
Annual Reports of the Victorian Department of Mental Hygiene,
    Department of Mental Health, Mental Hygiene Authority and
    Mental Health Authority, 1902–1978, in *Papers Presented to
    the Parliament* (Victoria)
Anon., 'After 20 Years', *Sun*, 16 July 1969
——'Case of the Substitute Salt', *Time*, 28 February 1949, p. 25
——'City Stops the Sale of Salt Substitute', *New York Times*,
    20 February 1949
——'4th Salt Product Branded As Poison', *New York Times*,
    1 March 1949
——'Freud's Theories Called "Blight on Minds of Men"', *Age*,
    8 May 1951
——'Fruiterer Stabbed: Woman Compatriot for Trial', *Argus*,
    31 August 1929

—'Help for the Manic-Depressive', *Time*, 20 April 1970, p. 42

—'Mental Health Doctor's Honor', *Brunswick Sentinel*,
28 January 1976

—'Salt Substitute Kills 4, AMA Says', *New York Times*,
19 February 1949

Ashburner, J.V., 'A case of chronic mania treated with lithium
citrate and terminating fatally', *Medical Journal of Australia*,
1950, vol. II: 386

The Australian and New Zealand Pharmaceutical Formulary,
7th edn, Melbourne, Pharmaceutical Association of Australia
and New Zealand, 1947 (1949 reprint)

Baastrup, P.C. and Schou, M., 'Lithium as a prophylactic agent:
Its effect against recurrent depressions and manic-depressive
psychosis', *Archives of General Psychiatry*, 1967, 16: 162–72

—'Prophylactic lithium', *Lancet*, 29 June 1968, 1419–22

Beaumont, Joan (ed.), *Australia's War, 1939–45*, Allen & Unwin:
Sydney, 1996

Berrios, G.E. and Freeman, H., *150 Years of British Psychiatry:
The aftermath*, Gaskell: London, 1996

Berrios, G.E. and Porter, R. (eds), *A History of Clinical Psychiatry:
The origin and history of psychiatric disorders*, Athlone Press:
London, 1995

Birch, H.M., 'Electrical convulsive therapy', *Medical Journal of
Australia*, 1942, 1: 675–8

Blackwell, B., 'Lithium: prophylactic or panacea?' *Medical
Counterpoint*, 1969, 11: 52–9

—'Need for careful evaluation of lithium', *American Journal of
Psychiatry*, 1969, 125: 1131

—'Lithium', *Lancet*, 24 October 1970, 875

—'Prophylactic lithium: Science or science fiction?' *American
Heart Journal*, 1972, 83: 139–41

—'The history of lithium therapy, by F.N. Johnson' (review),
Psychological Medicine, 1985, 15: 695–7

—'Bits and pieces of a psychiatrist's life', Xlibris Corporation,
2012

Blackwell, B. and Shepherd, M., 'Prophylactic lithium: Another therapeutic myth?', *Lancet*, 4 May 1968, 968–71

Bourne, H., 'The Insulin myth', *Lancet*, 7 November 1953, 964–8

Bowden, T., 'Changi photographer: George Aspinall's record of captivity', ABC/William Collins: Sydney, 1984

Burnet, F.M., Cade, J.F.J. and Lush, D., 'The serological response to influenza virus infection during an epidemic, with particular reference to subclinical infection', *Medical Journal of Australia*, 1940, vol. I, 397–401

Butler, A.G., *Official History of the Australian Army Medical Services 1914–1918*, vol. II, *The Western Front*, Australian War Memorial: Canberra, 1940

Cade J.F., 'John Frederick Joseph Cade: Family memories on the occasion of the 50th anniversary of his discovery of the use of lithium in mania', *Australian and New Zealand Journal of Psychiatry*, 1999, 33: 615–18

Cade, J.F.J., 'Death from arterial spasm', *Medical Journal of Australia*, 1938, vol. II: 168

——'A statistical study of the onset of primary dementia', *Medical Journal of Australia*, 1940, vol. II: 285–7

——'The anticonvulsant properties of creatinine', *Medical Journal of Australia*, 1947, vol. II: 621–3

——'Lithium salts in the treatment of psychotic excitement', *Medical Journal of Australia*, 1949, vol. II: 349–52

——'Insertion: Lithium treatment of mania', *Australasian Psychiatric Quarterly Newsletter*, 1949, vol. I (4)

——'Research in psychiatry: Beattie Smith Lecture I', *Medical Journal of Australia*, 1951, vol. II: 213–19

——'The problem of schizophrenia: Beattie Smith Lecture II', *Medical Journal of Australia*, 1951, vol. II: 245–51

——'The use of paraldehyde in alcoholic delirium tremens', *Medical Journal of Australia*, 1953, vol. II: 276–7

——'The aetiology of schizophrenia', *Medical Journal of Australia*, 1956, vol. II: 135–9

——'Alcoholism: A community responsibility', *Medical Journal of Australia*, 1956, vol. I: 363–6

——'Manganese and Mongolism', *Medical Journal of Australia*, 1958, vol. II: 848–9

——'Physical signs in clinical psychiatry', *Medical Journal of Australia*, 1961, vol. II: 994–6

——'The relation between recovery and plasma potassium levels in manic states', *Medical Journal of Australia*, 1962, vol. II: 911–13

——'A significant elevation of plasma magnesium levels in schizophrenia and depressive states', *Medical Journal of Australia*, 1964, vol. I: 195–6

——'The biochemistry of schizophrenic and affective psychoses', *Medical Journal of Australia*, 1964, vol. I: 878–81

——'The metabolism of melancholia', *Australian and New Zealand Journal of Psychiatry*, 1967, 1: 23–9

——'Obituary: Hedley Francis Summons', *Medical Journal of Australia*, 1967, vol. II: 87

——'Lithium in psychiatry: Historical origins and present position', *Australian and New Zealand Journal of Psychiatry*, 1967, 1: 61–2

——'The use of lithium salts in the treatment of mania', *Supplement to the Bulletin of the Post-Graduate Committee of Medicine, University of Sydney*, April 1969, pp. lxxiix–lxxxiii

——'The story of lithium', in Ayd, F.J. and Blackwell, B. (eds), *Discoveries in Biological Psychiatry*, J.B. Lippincott Co.: Philadelphia, PA, 1970, pp. 218–29

——'Contemporary challenges in psychiatry', *Australian and New Zealand Journal of Psychiatry*, 1971, 5: 10–17

——'Recent advances in the use of lithium', *Australian and New Zealand Journal of Psychiatry*, 1971, 5: 3–4

——'Massive thiamine dosage in the treatment of acute alcoholic psychoses', *Australian and New Zealand Journal of Psychiatry*, 1972, 6: 225–30

——'Masturbational madness: An historical annotation', *Australian and New Zealand Journal of Psychiatry*, 1973, 7: 23–6

——'An eclectic psychiatrist looks at homosexuality', in McConaghy, N. (ed.), *Liberation Movements and Psychiatry*, Geigy Psychiatric Symposium: Prince Henry Hospital, Ciba-Geigy: St Leonards, 1974, pp. 97–101

——'Lithium—when, why and how?' *Medical Journal of Australia*, 1975, vol. 1: 684–6

——'Lithium in medicine', in Burrows, G.D. and Chiu, E., *Research in Affective Disorders: Proceedings of the Scientific Meeting in Honour of Dr John F.J. Cade*, 4 February 1977, University of Melbourne: Melbourne, pp. 7–9

——'Lithium—past, present and future', in Johnson, F.N. and Johnson, S. (eds), *Lithium in medical practice: Proceedings of the First British Lithium Congress, University of Lancaster, England, 15–19 July 1977*, MTP Press: Lancaster, UK, 1978, pp. 5–16

——*Mending the Mind: A short history of twentieth century psychiatry*, Sun Books: Melbourne, 1979

Cade, J.F.J, articles written under the pseudonym 'Mensana', *The Messenger*, 1 September 1951 to 1 August 1952

Cade, J.F.J. and Krupinski J., 'Incidence of psychiatric disorders in Victoria in relation to country of birth', *Medical Journal of Australia*, 1962, vol. 1: 400–4

Cameron, A.T., *Recent Advances in Endocrinology*, J. & A. Churchill: London, 1945

Cawte, J., *The Last of the Lunatics*, Melbourne University Press: Melbourne, 1998

Cawte, J., 'Mania pre-lithium', *Australian and New Zealand Journal of Psychiatry*, 1999, 33: S7–S12

Chiu, E. and Hegarty, R.M., 'John Cade: The man', *Australian and New Zealand Journal of Psychiatry*, 1999, 33: S24–S26

Churchill, W.S., *History of the Second World War*, vol. 4, London, 1951

Conan Doyle, A., 'The Adventure of the Solitary Cyclist', in *The Return of Sherlock Holmes*, The Strand Magazine, 1904. Reproduced in *The Illustrated Sherlock Holmes Treasury*, Avenel Books: New York, 1976

Corcoran, A.C., Taylor, R.D. and Page, I.H., 'Lithium poisoning from the use of salt substitutes', *Journal of the American Medical Association*, 1949, 139: 685–8

Craig, D.A., *The Lion of Beechworth*, Specialty Press: Albury, 2000

Cramond, W.A., 'Lessons from the insulin story in psychiatry', *Australian and New Zealand Journal of Psychiatry*, 1987, 21: 320–6

Cunningham Dax, E., *Asylum to Community: The Development of the Mental Hygiene Service in Victoria, Australia*, F.W. Cheshire: Melbourne, 1961

Dane, P.G., 'Psycho-analysis', *Medical Journal of Australia*, 1949, vol II: 127–9

Davies, B., 'The first patient to receive lithium' (reprint), *The Australian and New Zealand Journal of Psychiatry*, 1999, 33: S32–S34

Dawson, W.S., *Aids to Psychiatry*, 3rd edn, Baillière, Tindall and Cox: London, 1934

Derham, A.P., 'Singapore and after: A brief historical survey of the activities of the Australian Army Medical Corps in Malaya', *Medical Journal of Australia*, 1946, vol II: 397–401

Ellard, J., McConaghy, N., Peterson, B., Cawte, J. and Grounds, D., 'Tributes to John Cade at the 50th anniversary dinner, Sydney, December 1999', *Australasian Psychiatry*, 2000, 8(2): 177–81

Ellery, R.S., *The Cow Jumped Over the Moon: Private papers of a psychiatrist*, F.W. Cheshire: Melbourne, 1956

Ellingsen, Peter, *A History of Psychoanalysis in Australia: From Freud to Lacan*, PsychOz Publications: Kew, Vic., 2013

Field, J.W., Green, R. and Byron, F.E., *The Institute for Medical Research Kuala Lumpur 1900–1950: Fifty years of medical research in Malaya*, Government Press: Kuala Lumpur, 1951

Fieve, Ronald, *Moodswing: The third revolution in psychiatry*, Bantam Books: New York, 1997

Garton, S., 'Changing Minds' in Curthoys A., Martin, A.W. and Rowse, T. (eds), *Australians from 1939*, Fairfax, Syme and Weldon Associates: Sydney, 1987

Gillies, Midge, *The Barbed-Wire University: The real lives of Allied POWs in the Second World War*, Aurum Press: London, 2011

Glesinger, B., 'Evaluation of lithium in treatment of psychotic excitement', *Medical Journal of Australia*, 1954, vol I: 277–83

Goodwin, F.K., Murphy, D.L. and Bunney, W.E., 'Lithium', *Lancet*, 26 July 1969, 212–13

Gregory, A.T., 'Jewels in the crown: *The Medical Journal of Australia*'s 10 most-cited articles', *Medical Journal of Australia*, 2004, 181: 9–12.

Grob, G.N., 'Psychiatry's Holy Grail: The search for the mechanisms of mental diseases', *Bulletin of the History of Medicine*, 1998, 72: 189–219

Haigh, G., 'Matter over mind', *The Bulletin*, 21 December 2004–11 January 2005, pp. 91–5

Hanlon, L.W., Romaine, M., Gilroy, F.J., et al., 'Lithium chloride as a substitute for sodium chloride in the diet', *Journal of the American Medical Association*, 1949, 139(11): 688–92

Healy, David, *The Creation of Psychopharmacology*, Harvard University Press: Cambridge, MA, 2002

Hearder, R., *Keep the Men Alive*, Allen & Unwin: Sydney, 2009

Jamison, K.R., *An Unquiet Mind*, Alfred A. Knopf: New York, 1995

Johnson, Carl, *Carrying on Under Fire and in Captivity: Stories from the 8th Division Australian Army Medical Corps under Malaya command*, History House: Melbourne, 2009

Johnson, F.N., 'John F.J. Cade, 1912 to 1980: A reminiscence', *Pharmacopsychiatria*, 1981, 14: 148–9

——*The History of Lithium Therapy*, Macmillan: London, 1984

Johnson, F.N. and Cade, J.F.J., 'The historical background to lithium research and therapy', in Johnson, F.N. (ed.), *Lithium Research and Therapy*, Academic Press: London, 1975, pp. 9–22

Kennedy, Alexander, 'Report to the Minister for Health on Mental Health and Mental Hygiene Services in the State of Victoria:

1 January, 1950', Victorian Government Printer: Department of Health, Melbourne, 1950

Kirschner, M.W., Marincola, E. and Teisberg, E.O., 'The role of biomedical research in health care reform', *Science*, 1994, 266: 49–51

Kraepelin, E., *Dementia Praecox and Paraphrenia together with Manic-Depressive Insanity and Paranoia*, Classics of Medicine Library: Birmingham, 1989

Krupinski J., Schaechter F. and Cade J.F.J., 'Factors influencing the incidence of mental disorders among migrants', *Medical Journal of Australia*, 1965, vol. II: 269–77

Likeman, R., *Men of the Ninth: A history of the Ninth Australian Field Ambulance, 1916–1994*, Slouch Hat Publications: McCrae, Vic, 2003

Lowe, J., 'I don't believe in God, but I believe in lithium', *New York Times Magazine*, 25 June 2015

McLachlan, Iaen, 'Doctor Reports on: New methods of treating mentally ill', *Age*, 20 August 1954

McPhee, Peter, *'Pansy': A life of Roy Douglas Wright*, Melbourne University Press: Melbourne, 1999

Marks, Harry M., *The Progress of Experiment: Science and therapeutic reform in the United States, 1900–1990*, Cambridge University Press: Cambridge, NY, 1997

Martindale, *The Extra Pharmacopoeia*, vol. 1, 22nd edn, Council of the Pharmaceutical Society of Great Britain: London, 1941

Melia, P.I., 'Lithium', *Lancet*, 26 April 1969, 889–90

Noack, C.H. and Trautner, E.M., 'The lithium treatment of maniacal psychosis', *Medical Journal of Australia*, 1951, vol. II: 219–22

Odgers, G., 'Can we ignore this Xmas challenge?' *Argus*, 15 December 1953

Rank, Benjamin K., *The Family Story: A mirror of shared inheritance*, Brolga Press: Canberra, 1992

Richards, R., *A Doctor's War*, HarperCollins Publishers: Sydney, 2005

Roberts, E.L., 'A case of chronic mania treated with lithium citrate and terminating fatally', *Medical Journal of Australia*, 1950, vol. II: 261–2

Rodgers, Joann, 'From fireworks, a substantially safe element: Strontium carbonate may help mentally depressed', *News American*, 20 April 1970

Ross, R., 'New key to mental health', *Australian Women's Weekly*, 13 May 1970

Safe, M., 'A beautiful mind', *Weekend Australian Magazine*, 2–3 October 2004, pp. 28–9

Schioldann, J., *History of the Introduction of Lithium into Medicine and Psychiatry: Birth of Modern Psychopharmacology 1949*, Adelaide: Adelaide Academic Press/Brascoe Publishing, 2009

Schou, M., Juel-Nielsen, N., Strömgren E. and Voldby, H., 'The treatment of manic psychoses by the administration of lithium salts', *Journal of Neurology, Neurosurgery & Psychiatry*, 1954, 17: 250–60

Schou, M., 'The early European lithium studies', *Australian and New Zealand Journal of Psychiatry*, 1999, 33: S39–S47

Scottish Medico-Psychological Association, *Handbook for Mental Nurses*, 7th edn, London: Baillière, Tindall and Cox, 1941 [1885]

Seal, R. Eric., 'An emerging dimension in psychiatry—From depth to height', in Chiu, Edmond (ed.), *Psychiatry and Religion: Proceedings of a conference*, 27–28 June 1985, St Vincent's Hospital, Melbourne

Sharpe, David and Sharpe, Kathleen E., *Pharmacy Families: Henry Francis in Australia 1849–1999*, Cossar: Melbourne, 1999

Shephard, B., *A War of Nerves: Soldiers and psychiatrists 1914–1994*, Pimlico: London, 2002

——'A prophylactic myth', *International Journal of Psychiatry*, 1971, 9: 423–5

——'Review of: "Neil Johnson: The history of lithium therapy"', Macmillan: London, 1984, *Medical History*, 1985, 29: 223–4

Shorter, Edward, *A History of Psychiatry: From the era of the asylum to the Age of Prozac*, John Wiley & Sons: New York, 1997

Smith, Dean A. and Woodruff, Michael F.A., *Deficiency Diseases in Japanese Prison Camps*, London, UK Medical Research Medical Council, No. 274, Special Report Series, 1951

Squire, Peter, *Companion to the British Pharmacopoeia*, 19th edn, Churchill: London, 1916

Stern, R.L., 'Severe lithium chloride poisoning with complete recovery: Report of case', *Journal of the American Medical Association*, 1949, 139(11): 710–11

Stoller, A., 'Lithium therapy of chronic mania', *Australasian Psychiatric Quarterly Newsletter*, 1950, 2: 10

Trautner, E.M., Morris, R., Noack, C.H. and Gershon, S., 'The excretion and retention of ingested lithium and its effect on the ionic balance of man', *Medical Journal of Australia*, 1955, vol. II: 280–91

Wells, H.G., 'The Reconciliation', in *H.G. Wells Short Stories*, Folio Society: London, 1990

Westmore, Ann, Entry on 'John Cade', in Bynum, William F. and Bynum, Helen (eds), *Dictionary of Medical Biography*, vol. 2, C–G, Greenwood: Westport, CT, London, 2007, pp. 290–1

——'Eric Cunningham Dax: A tribute', *Health and History*, 2008, 10(1): 167–71

——'The many faces of John Cade' (Appendix II), in Schioldann, Johan, *History of the Introduction of Lithium into Medicine and Psychiatry: Birth of modern psychopharmacology 1949*, Adelaide Academic Press: Adelaide, 2009, 309–12

Westmore, Ann and de Moore, Greg, 'The mad major and his idiosyncratic war: Linking military medicine and lithium therapy for mania', *Health and History*, 2013, 15(1): 11–37

Westmore, Ann and Weisz, George M., 'Medical research undertaken in captivity: A form of resistance to imprisonment and attempted extermination', *War & Society*, 2009, 28(1): 89–112

White, J. Glyn, 'Administrative and clinical problems in Australian and British prisoner-of-war camps in Singapore, 1942 to 1945', *Medical Journal of Australia*, 1946, vol. II: 401–3

Wiles, Jo, 'Dr John's prostitute was moral to psychiatry staff', *Age*, 22 January 1977

Wilkinson, G. (ed.), *Talking About Psychiatry*, London: Gaskell, 1993

Willingham, Allan, *Bundoora Park (J.V. Smith Homestead): A cultural history and conservation plan*, Melbourne: Allan Willingham, 1996

Woodruff, Michael F.A., *Nothing Venture Nothing Win*, Edinburgh: Scottish Academic Press, 1996

Wright, R.D., 'What Australian physiology owes to Adolph Hitler', *Proceedings of The Australian Physiological and Pharmacological Society*, 1983, 14(1): 22–7

Unpublished sources

Cade, David D., 'Memoir', written c. 1945 (Cade family papers)

Cade, David Jnr, written memories of his father, Dr John Cade and his family (2011)

Cade, J.F.J., Academic record, University of Melbourne Archives

——Lecture given on 11 May 1978, 'Psychiatry in Changi Prison: three and a half years on the receiving end in a POW camp' (Cade family papers)

——Letters to Jean Cade before, during and immediately after World War II (Cade family papers)

——'Memoirs of the mad major', undated manuscript written in the late 1970s and covering the period early 1930s to 1941 (Cade family papers)

——Miscellaneous items and letters and memorabilia kept by the four Cade boys. This includes their father's books—*Malay Vocabulary* from Changi, and his copy of *Rats, Lice and History*. It includes the American Psychiatric Association pamphlet, including Cade's handwritten speech, his papers on Freud, and various newsletters of the 2/9th Field Ambulance

——Notes for lectures given to medical and psychology students
(Ed Chiu papers)

Cade, John and Jean, Letters to family members during trip to
examine British psychiatry, 1954 (Cade family papers)

Elder, David, 'Notes on Brushes with the British over Medical
Arrangements', undated, provided by David Elder to Ann
Westmore, 20 November 2001

Hearder, Rosalind, 'Careers in Captivity: Australian POW Medical
Officers in Japanese Captivity During WW II', PhD thesis,
University of Melbourne, 2003

Hill, David, 'Notes on lecture given by John Cade during 1960s'

Jones, W. Ernest, memoirs written c. 1939, Royal Melbourne
Hospital archives

Lugton, Don, 'Reflections on John Cade by Members of his Unit',
undated document provided by Bill Flowers to Ann Westmore,
18 February 1999

Minute book of the Mental Hygiene Medical Officers' Association,
Victorian Department of Human Services Mental Health
Archive, Royal Melbourne Hospital

Noone, Val, 'Notes on lecture given by John Cade during 1960s'

Westmore, Ann, 'Mind, Mania and Science: Psychiatry and the
culture of experiment in mid-twentieth century Victoria', PhD
thesis, University of Melbourne, 2002

About the authors

GREG DE MOORE is an Associate Professor of Psychiatry based at Sydney's Westmead Hospital. Born in Melbourne of parents who migrated to Australia from Sri Lanka, Greg has lived in Sydney for over 30 years. Outside of the hospital he has combined his medical interests with Australian history to write and co-write two previous books—*Tom Wills* and *A National Game*. The biography of Tom Wills was based on ten years of research unearthing original medical records, letters, textbooks and notes previously believed to have been lost or destroyed. This book won numerous awards and was shortlisted for the National Biography Award. Greg has also written on the need to preserve psychiatric records as a precious storehouse of clinical and social history.

ANN WESTMORE is an Honorary Fellow in the Health Humanities and Social Science Unit, School of Population and Global Health, at the University of Melbourne. She came to the history of medicine and science through a degree in science and a previous career as a medical writer for a mass circulation newspaper. After completing a Master of Science in the history and philosophy of science, Ann completed a PhD titled 'Mind, Mania and Science: Psychiatry and the Culture of Experiment in Mid-Twentieth Century Victoria'. Her thesis gave rise to work with Museum Victoria and the University of Melbourne investigating nineteenth and twentieth century mental health care in Australia. In 2010 she commenced work with Greg de Moore on a biography of John Cade while also working on a history of psychiatry in Victoria in the twentieth century.

Index

Page numbers in *italic* refer to photographs

Index